MARGIN CONTROL SURGERY OF THE SKIN
Concepts, Histopathology, and Applications

Patrick Emanuel, MB, ChB, FRCPA
Dermatopathologist
Clinica Ricardo Palma
San Isidro, Lima, Peru
Consultant Dermatopathologist
Pathlab Bay of Plenty, Tauranga, New Zealand
Honorary Associate Professor
Department of Pathology and Molecular Medicine
University of Auckland
Auckland, New Zealand
Adjunct Assistant Professor
Department of Dermatology, Mount Sinai Hospital
New York, New York

Mark Izzard, MBBS, FRACS
Otolaryngologist, Head and Neck Surgeon
Director
Micro-Vascular Reconstructive Surgeon
Auckland Head and Neck Specialists
Director
Skin Institute, New Zealand
Senior Lecturer
ORL Head and Neck Surgery
University of Auckland
Auckland, New Zealand

New York   Chicago   San Francisco   Athens   London   Madrid   Mexico City
Milan   New Delhi   Singapore   Sydney   Toronto

Margin Control Surgery of the Skin: Concepts, Histopathology, and Applications

1 2 3 4 5 6 7 8 9 DSS 28 27 26 25 24 23

ISBN 978-1-264-28599-0
MHID 1-264-28599-X

NOTICE

Medicine is an ever-changing science. As new research and clinical experience broaden our knowledge, changes in treatment and drug therapy are required. The author and the publisher of this work have checked with sources believed to be reliable in their efforts to provide information that is complete and generally in accord with the standards accepted at the time of publication. However, in view of the possibility of human error or changes in medical sciences, neither the author nor the publisher nor any other party who has been involved in the preparation or publication of this work warrants that the information contained herein is in every respect accurate or complete, and they disclaim all responsibility for any errors or omissions or for the results obtained from use of the information contained in this work. Readers are encouraged to confirm the information contained herein with other sources. For example and in particular, readers are advised to check the product information sheet included in the package of each drug they plan to administer to be certain that the information contained in this work is accurate and that changes have not been made in the recommended dose or in the contraindications for administration. This recommendation is of particular importance in connection with new or infrequently used drugs.

This book was set in Minion Pro by MPS Limited.
The editors were Dimana Tzvetkova and Kim J. Davis.
The production supervisor was Richard Ruzycka.
Project management was provided by Alok Singh of MPS Limited.
The cover designer was W2 Design.

This book is printed on acid-free paper.

Library of Congress Cataloging-in-Publication Data

Names: Emanuel, Patrick, editor. | Izzard, Mark, editor.
Title: Margin control surgery of the skin : concepts, histopathology,
   and applications / [edited by] Patrick Emanuel, Mark Izzard.
Description: New York : McGraw Hill LLC, [2023] | Includes bibliographical references and index.
Identifiers: LCCN 2022048655 (print) | LCCN 2022048656 (ebook) |
   ISBN 9781264285990 (paperback; alk. paper) | ISBN 9781264285983 (ebook)
Subjects: MESH: Skin Neoplasms—surgery | Margins of Excision | Skin Neoplasms—pathology |
   Dermatologic Surgical Procedures—methods | Specimen Handling—methods
Classification: LCC RD520 (print) | LCC RD520 (ebook) | NLM WR 500 |
   DDC 617.4/77—dc23/eng/20230203
LC record available at https://lccn.loc.gov/2022048655
LC ebook record available at https://lccn.loc.gov/2022048656

McGraw Hill books are available at special quantity discounts to use as premiums and sales promotions or for use in corporate training programs. To contact a representative, please visit the Contact Us pages at www.mhprofessional.com.

MARGIN CONTROL SURGERY OF THE SKIN

Concepts, Histopathology, and Applications

This book is dedicated to:

Claudia, Diego, Simon, Laura
—Patrick

Ro, Sean, Issy, Liv, Peri, Lili
—Mark

Contents

Contributors ix
Preface xi
Acknowledgments xiii
Introduction xv

SECTION I: Background 1

1. **History** 3
   Patrick Emanuel, Victor Brodsky

2. **Multidisciplinary Approach** 9
   Patrick Emanuel, Rajan S. Patel

3. **Mohs Micrographic Surgery** 17
   Rebecca Kleinerman, Patrick Emanuel

**SECTION II: Surgical Considerations, Specimen Preparation,
and Processing** 27

4. **Indications** 29
   Patrick Emanuel, Kevin G. Smith

5. **Surgical Technique and Specimen Mapping** 35
   Mark Izzard, Patrick Emanuel

6. **Specimen Preparation** 53
   Patrick Emanuel, Mark Izzard

7. **Slide Preparation and Immunohistochemistry** 77
   Patrick Emanuel, Martin Cavanagh

SECTION III: Applications for Cutaneous Malignancy 89

8. **Basal Cell Carcinoma** 91
   Patrick Emanuel, Mark Izzard

9. **Cutaneous Squamous Cell Carcinoma** 111
   Patrick Emanuel, Garrett Desman

10. **Melanoma** 127
    Patrick Emanuel, Gonzalo Ziegler-Rodriguez

11. **Cutaneous Sarcomas**.. 147
    Patrick Emanuel, Mauricio León Rivera

12. **Merkel Cell Carcinoma** 165
    Patrick Emanuel, Mark Izzard

13. **Malignant Adnexal Tumors** 175
    Patrick Emanuel, Mark Izzard

14. **Extramammary Paget's Disease**.. 195
    Richard B. Johnston, Patrick Emanuel

SECTION IV: Case Reports and Discussions.. 201

15. **Case 1. Basic Basal Cell Carcinoma**... 203
    Patrick Emanuel, Mark Izzard

16. **Case 2. Large Facial Lentigo Maligna** 211
    Patrick Emanuel, Mark Izzard

17. **Case 3. Microcystic Adnexal Carcinoma**... 217
    Patrick Emanuel, Mark Izzard

18. **Case 4. Dermatofibrosarcoma Protuberans of the Scalp**............................ 223
    Patrick Emanuel, Mark Izzard

19. **Case 5. Pleomorphic Dermal Sarcoma of the Scalp** 231
    Patrick Emanuel, Mark Izzard, Edgar Jesus Salas Moscoso

Index 235

Contributors

Victor Brodsky, MD
Associate Professor of Pathology and Immunology
Associate Medical Director of Information Systems
School of Medicine
Washington University in St. Louis
St. Louis, Missouri

Martin Cavanagh, QMLT Histology
Skin Institute Ltd
Auckland, New Zealand

Garrett Desman, MD
Chief of Dermatopathology Services
Optum Tri-State
Assistant Clinical Professor of Pathology & Dermatology
Icahn School of Medicine at Mount Sinai
New York, New York

Patrick Emanuel, MB, ChB, FRCPA
Dermatopathologist
Clinica Ricardo Palma
San Isidro, Lima, Peru
Consultant Dermatopathologist
Pathlab Bay of Plenty, Tauranga, New Zealand
Honorary Associate Professor
Department of Pathology and Molecular Medicine
University of Auckland
Auckland, New Zealand
Adjunct Assistant Professor, Department of Dermatology
Mount Sinai Hospital
New York, New York

Mark Izzard, MBBS, FRACS
Otolaryngologist, Head and Neck Surgeon
Director
Micro-Vascular Reconstructive Surgeon
Auckland Head and Neck Specialists
Director
Skin Institute, New Zealand
Senior Lecturer
ORL Head and Neck Surgery
Auckland University
Auckland, New Zealand

Richard B. Johnston, MBChB, PhD
Fred Hutchinson Cancer Research Institute
Seattle, Washington

Rebecca Kleinerman, MD
Private Practice, Dermatology
Clinical Instructor, Mount Sinai Hospital
New York, New York

Edgar Jesus Salas Moscoso, MD, MeB
Head and Neck Surgery and Oncology
Minimally Invasive and Robotic Head and Neck Surgery
Ricardo Palma Clinic
Lima, Peru

Rajan S. Patel, MBChB, MD, FRCS, FRACS
Head & Neck, Facial Plastics & Reconstructive Surgeon
Skin Institute and MercyAscot Hospitals
Auckland, New Zealand

Mauricio León Rivera, MD
Professor of Oncological Surgery of Skin, Breast, and Soft Tissue Tumors
Universidad Peruana de Ciencias Aplicadas
Lima, Peru

Kevin G. Smith, MA, MBBS, FRACS (OHNS)
Clinical Lead for Head & Neck Surgery
Waitemata Health
Auckland, New Zealand

Gonzalo Ziegler-Rodriguez, MD, FACS
Surgical Oncologist
Chief, Melanoma and Skin Cancer Unit
Clinica Ziegler
Lima, Peru

Preface

The primary goal of this book is to explain what cutaneous margin control surgery (MCS) is and how you can apply it to your skin cancer surgery or pathology practice. We'll explain why it is needed, what options exist for how to perform it, and the scenarios it can be applied in. Hopefully, those already doing MCS will learn some new concepts, techniques, and applications. We set ourselves the lofty goal of writing a text which can be read with ease from cover to cover while hopefully still being interesting and accurate. To avoid going off on unnecessary tangents and to limit repetition, we've aimed for cohesion by being involved in all the chapters while still benefiting from the expertise of the invited contributing authors.

We've used acronyms in the text. Though these can be distracting, we ultimately decided to mimic most contemporary texts by using those that are widely known for the sake of consistency. We've limited them to those we think are essential and encourage the reader to familiarize themselves with these.

In the recommendations put out by the National Comprehensive Cancer Network® (NCCN), MCS is included as a treatment option for a variety of skin cancers. For one set of tumors, MCS is suggested as an alternative to a standard surgical excision with the recommended measured surgical margins (e.g., high-risk squamous cell carcinoma [SCC] and basal cell carcinoma [BCC]). For another set of tumors, MCS is recommended as the only surgical option (e.g., dermatofibrosarcoma protuberans), while for a different set of tumors, MCS is recommended but for specific scenarios (e.g., melanoma *in situ* or minimally invasive melanoma on cosmetically sensitive skin).

Mohs micrographic surgery (MMS) or continuous complete peripheral and deep margin assessment (CCPDMA; also called peripheral and deep *en face* margin assessment [PDEMA]) is practically equivalent therapies in the NCCN. There are numerous textbooks, training programs, societies, and annual conferences for MMS. But what is CCPDMA? Is it the same thing done by a different type of specialist? Is it something new?

CCPDMA involves the examination of the entire peripheral and deep margin without any gaps. In the NCCN definition, a surgical procedure can be described as CCPDMA if all the following criteria are met:

- The entire marginal surface is microscopically examined.
- The surgical specimen is orientated so that a positive margin can be mapped.
- The surgical margin is re-excised and once more the entire margin is visualized until a clear margin is assured.
- The steps are rapid enough to ensure no significant change in the size of the wound.

CCPDMA can be achieved with histopathologic examination using intraoperative frozen section processing or with formalin-fixed paraffin processing. There are a variety of laboratory methods available to achieve this goal. Just as there are no studies to compare variations of the MMS techniques, there is no evidence to suggest that the different forms of MCS (MMS or CCPDMA) have different cure rates. Common sense would agree with the NCCN in considering the MCS options as equivalent procedures.

There are many mentions in the literature of the superior cure rates of MCS when compared with a "wide local excision." But any comparison depends entirely on how the specimen has been processed in the laboratory and the consequent thoroughness of the margin assessment.

A whole range of medical professionals excises skin cancers. Plastic and reconstructive surgeons, dermatologists, head and neck surgeons, general surgeons, and general practitioners do so in their daily practice. Rather than engaging in some form of surgical *paragone* or debate as to which type of doctor is best equipped to achieve negative surgical margins, we hope this text interests *all* types of surgeons as they strive for the best surgical results for their patients.

To cater to this wider audience, we've focused mainly on common tumors and scenarios. However, we've also attempted to show that some of the techniques can be applied to the treatment of more advanced or uncommon malignancies usually dealt with by oncologic surgeons rather than dermatologists or primary care doctors with an interest in skin cancer.

Pathologists and laboratory staff are usually charged with the task of assessing the margins of skin excisions. They may be well-versed in some techniques but less familiar with some of the other options or perhaps uncomfortable with their use for certain tumors. We hope this book clears up some of these concerns.

An understanding of the histopathology of skin tumors helps in formulating a surgical strategy. Throughout the book, we've integrated the relevant pathology and some of the key issues that need to be considered for the various tumors. We hope this will be of interest to surgeons as well as pathologists. One reason why MMS has proved so successful is that the operating surgeon understands and usually interprets the pathology. This understanding is, however, not beyond the scope of other surgeons, especially those who work closely with their colleagues in pathology.

Where possible, histopathologic photos of frozen section slides are used to illustrate features. While this means the images are not as clear as those from paraffin-embedded tissue, we believe these more accurately reflect what is seen in routine practice.

Finally, we've tried to create a text which encourages a sense of collegiality. An integrated collegial approach in which specialties learn from each other serves the patient well and is to be encouraged above other more mundane considerations. Collegiality is equally important in all geographic locations, regardless of the access that patients have to different specialist providers.

Patrick Emanuel, MB, ChB, FRCPA
Mark Izzard, MBBS, FRACS

Acknowledgments

Hone Johnson (Rotorua) made substantial contributions. He revised and corrected the text and captions, correcting all too numerous *orthographic innovations*.

Most of the histological slides were prepared in the dermatopathology laboratories of the Auckland District Health Board (New Zealand), Skin Institute (New Zealand), Clinica Ricardo Palma (Peru), and the Mount Sinai Medical Center (USA). We particularly wish to acknowledge the quality manager and histotechnologist at the Skin Institute, Colleen Bauckham, QMLT (Auckland) for her help in locating slides, and patient details.

The nursing staff at the Skin Institute helped organize the material and facilitated the process of patient consent. A special thanks to Priscilla Edgecombe-Macduff, RN for her help in creating a clinical environment in which high-quality care and innovation are achievable. Such an environment is essential and frequently overlooked.

We thank the patients who kindly consented for their photographs to appear in the book.

Introduction

Margins
Clinical Margin Assessment
How Large Should the Margin Be?

Mathematics
Skin Tumors Are Like Volcanoes, and Here's
  Why

MARGINS

The central goal of all skin cancer surgery is a complete tumor excision with the least possible morbidity. This seems like a simple goal, but the way *margins* are discussed can be confusing. Take for example Merkel cell carcinoma, for which a 1- to 3-cm excision margin is recommended. Does this mean 1 cm or 3 cm? Somewhere in the middle? Does it mean the preoperative clinical margin? Or is it the intraoperative margin? Histopathological margin? How are these margins different and what do they imply about the certainty that no tumor has been left behind?

Before tackling these questions, let us first consider the relatively basic tools most surgeons use to guide their skin cancer surgery.

CLINICAL MARGIN ASSESSMENT

Assessment of clinical margins is often the first step in any skin cancer excision. This entails a sort of mystical guesswork as to what lies beneath the surface based on prior experience, usually accompanied by a bit of a gut feeling combined with actual feeling or palpation of the lesion to be excised. The surgical marker is then put to work and the surgeon starts to draw. Most surgeons would struggle to remember if anyone taught them how to draw margins or if it was learned by osmosis, just watching it done by others. Like the famous joke of a man stopping a stranger in the street and asking, "How would you get to the pub from here?," the answer to which is, "if I was going to the pub I wouldn't start from here," where we start to draw the margin is not often discussed and is poorly described in the literature. It naturally depends on what sort of tumor we are dealing with, and why a preoperative biopsy is so important. Some tumors are easy to spot and grow in a regular fashion with a nice cohesive advancing tumor front. They do not often exhibit perineural invasion or lymphovascular invasion and hence often what you see is what you get. But other tumors are highly unpredictable and the invasive fronts extend in different directions in a seemingly chaotic fashion. For these tumors, the surgeon is basically *guessing* when they decide on the shape and size of the excision.

HOW LARGE SHOULD THE MARGIN BE?

As soon as you cut out the tumor, that clinical margin becomes a surgical or excision margin and there is an expected rim of "excess" tissue that is removed as a buffer zone around the tumor. Confusingly, there are a variety of guidelines defining how wide the clinical buffer zone needs to be. Let us take high-risk basal cell carcinoma (BCC) as an example. Any literature search will come up with 3 to 4 mm as an adequate excision margin for a low-risk lesion, but guidelines vary wildly for a high-risk lesion. The British Association of Dermatology specifies 5 to 13 mm but does not really say whether you should be nearer the 5 mm or the 13 mm. By contrast, the Australian Cancer Network considers this somewhat excessive and only stipulates 3 to 5 mm. The European Forum of Dermatology suggests 5 to 10 mm, which sits nicely between these two (**Table I.1**). Unless the BCCs are different in Australia, that's quite a disparity. But none of them describe how to *actually* draw this margin. Is the measurement taken from the outside of the very last bit of erythema and vasculature that you can see with your +2 glasses on? Or via reflectance confocal microscopy? Or is it a line drawn around the bulk of the obvious clinical tumor with a margin then added on to that? Even with the most sophisticated aids, it can be difficult to see tumor, and often we are looking at vasculature or other surrogate signs.

It's all rather unsatisfactory, which is of course why it's all so inconsistent in the literature. It's a big heterogeneous group of tumors and a big heterogenous group of surgeons trying to hammer square pegs into round holes. And while the surgeons are busy reading guidelines and drawing lines, the pathologists are using their graticules (a microscope eyepiece with an inbuilt ruler) to measure microscopic distances. These measurements produce a pathology report with seemingly magically concrete numbers and affirmations about margin status. But when you think a little deeper, it's clear that pathologic margin measurements can be even less precise than the clinical estimates.

MATHEMATICS

What this really boils down to is math, and if you're reading this book there's a good chance you were either good at math *or* good at biology, but maybe not both. It's possible you are not the former, but you are sure to understand that it's all to do with confidence intervals. A confidence interval is a range of values that's likely to include a value with a certain degree of confidence, often expressed as a percentage. In the skin surgery context, an increasing size of the excision margin results in a progressive decrease in the percentage of incomplete excisions. Importantly, even with very large excisions, a small percentage of tumors will involve the surgical margins.

TABLE I.1 Comparison of Margin Guidelines	
Organization	Peripheral Margins for High-Risk BCC
NCCN	>4 mm
EDF	5-10 mm
BAD	>5 mm
CCA/ACN	3-5 mm
Sweden	>5 mm

BAD, British Association of Dermatology; CCA/CAN, Cancer Council Australia and Australian Cancer Network; EDF, European Dermatology Forum; NCCN, National Cancer Care Network.

Let's imagine that you perform the mystical 5-mm surgical margin (presuming you know exactly where to start). This 5 mm is a surrogate for a lot of very complicated concepts hidden in the measurement such as the tumor biology, the growth patterns, the anatomic site of tumor, the tissue it's growing in, the state of the immune system of the host, and so on. The margin in this sense, i.e., the strip of normal-looking tissue that's removed in excess of the assessed tumor size, describes the confidence with which you will achieve complete tumor clearance. That strip of tissue may or may not contain tumor. As mentioned earlier, this depends on many factors, not least of which is how good the surgeon is at assessing clinically the extent of the tumor.

Margin guidelines are thus established with the understanding that a significant percentage of tumors will extend microscopically further than the recommendation. In essence, those who set margin guidelines are making a judgment call as to what percentage of incomplete tumor resections (outliers) is *acceptable*. According to the National Comprehensive Cancer Network® (NCCN), a 4-mm margin will remove a BCC 94% of the time. Stop to think about that. We wouldn't accept it if planes landed safely only 94% of the time. Considering that there are 3.5 million BCCs a year in the United States, and let's say that 75% are low risk, that's at least 150,000 people a year with a positive margin. So, in that case, would taking 5 mm be better, or 6 mm, or 10 mm? What's the impact on both morbidity and quality of life of taking larger margins? This is something that isn't discussed much in the literature: The true cost of recurrence versus the cost of excess margin.

SKIN TUMORS ARE LIKE VOLCANOES, AND HERE'S WHY

If you've ever visited New Zealand, you'd have noticed that there are volcanoes everywhere. Volcanoes in many other parts of the world have been worn down by erosion over the millennia and aren't nearly as exciting as Mount Taranaki. Every flight from the South Island of New Zealand up to Auckland in the North Island flies over it. This impressive and, in some ways, the otherworldly natural phenomenon can lead you to think about margins (**Fig. I.1**).

In the mind's eye, skin tumors are a lot like volcanoes, in that the clinical assessment determines where the edge of the slope meets the ground. Where does the volcano start and stop? From the side, Mt Taranaki looks very regular and smooth. But take a look at the satellite view from above (**Fig. I.2**).

The clinical disease is the snow-capped peak and the gentle slope of the classic volcano, but we can see subclinical areas of disease, at 11 o'clock. It's pretty hard to draw a uniform margin around the whole thing. At 11 o'clock we're getting pretty close to an important structure, the sea!

The **clinical** margin is the outline of the tumor we can see or *guess*.

The **surgical** margin is the excess we draw around our clinical margin.

The **excision** margin is what we actually remove, which correlates with the **pathological** margin, which is how far from the tumor our excision margin is (**Fig. I.3**).

We may use a dermatoscope to help define our clinical margins and aid us in the removal of the first excision level. Making dots on the skin as reference points and then going back and forth with the dermatoscope helps us to build up a picture of the tumor. But this is still *guesswork*, and a central theme of this book is to avoid *guesswork* as much as possible.

Therefore, what we need is a satellite image of the tumor-like Mt Taranaki. If we had a method to draw accurate clinical margins every time, we could thus achieve complete tumor clearance every time. Unfortunately, this is not something we have, and even the

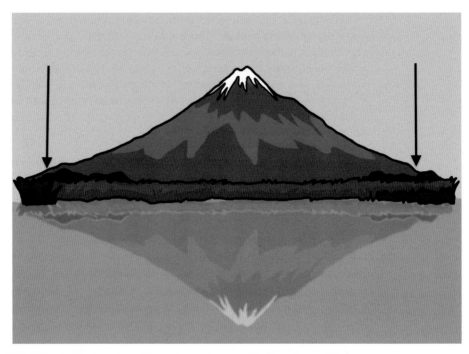

FIGURE I.1. **Is this the edge of the volcano? (arrows)** What's underneath?

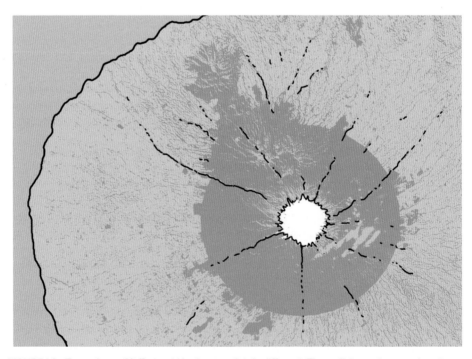

FIGURE I.2. **From above, Mt Taranaki looks completely different.** The radial margin spreads out irregularly at 11 o'clock.

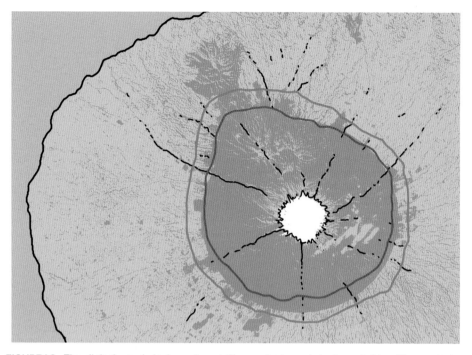

FIGURE I.3. **The clinical margin is drawn in red. The surgical margin is drawn in blue.** The surgical margin is only as good as the clinical margin.

latest imaging technologies cannot show us the detail we need to achieve this goal. We, therefore, need to turn to something else, something that is an afterthought for most surgeons: the pathologist. With a map.

If we could survey the tumor in real time, map the outside like a cartographer, every nook and cranny, every lahar and lava flow, we could build up a real-time 2D image of the tumor. A sort of satellite image from above. But this is only half the story. We need a Geotechnical engineer to do core samples across the entire area to assess its depth, shape, and the way it interacts with the surrounding structures.

In this analogy, the cartographer and Geotechnical engineer are the pathologist, and the technique used is referred to as margin control surgery (MCS). Terminology can get a little confusing as different specialties have different names for similar procedures. But the essential point is that, central to the concept of MCS, the *entire* surgical margin is assessed histopathologically, and this assessment guides the size and shape of the excision to achieve the complete removal of a tumor. Clinical *guesswork* is eliminated.

Once you've used and become accustomed to this assistance in surgery, it's like a lightbulb going on. And once you've seen the light, you won't want to go back into the gloom.

MARGIN CONTROL SURGERY OF THE SKIN

Concepts, Histopathology, and Applications

SECTION I
Background

History

Patrick Emanuel / Victor Brodsky

Early Attempts at Intraoperative Diagnoses
Frozen Section Pathology Is Invented
Frozen Section Pathology Becomes Widely
 Used

Intraoperative Margin Assessment in Cutaneous
 Surgery
An Entire Field Is Born
Final Thoughts

It is interesting to contemplate how differently margin assessment techniques might have evolved had it not been for a few key people. Who knows, perhaps instead of freezing and finely slicing tissue for margin assessment, we would be scanning tumors using some less-accurate imaging technology. Or maybe we would be diving straight into some form of costly and difficult molecular assessment.

EARLY ATTEMPTS AT INTRAOPERATIVE DIAGNOSES

In the 19th century, many surgeons examined tumors macroscopically themselves. By today's standards, this was crude, but it did serve some purpose in trying to determine whether a lesion was malignant. The specimen was often disposed of afterward without much in the way of documentation or a formal diagnosis. The introduction of methods of fixation, the microtome (an instrument that finely cuts tissues to prepare microscopic slides), and microscopy paved the way for surgical pathology. Rudolf Virchow (1821-1902) is generally recognized as the father of microscopic pathology. An innovative polymath, he was known by his colleagues at Berlin's Charité Hospital as "The Pope" due to his authority and influence. Due in no small part to his contributions, surgical pathology expanded from a purely macroscopic examination performed by surgeons to become the enormously important specialized medical field it continues to be today.[1-3]

FROZEN SECTION PATHOLOGY IS INVENTED

The invention of the frozen section can be traced back to various vague descriptions of assessments of fresh tissue using a microscope in the 1800s, and then more concise descriptions in the early 1900s.

In the Virchow laboratory, Julius Cohnheim pioneered the use of the frozen section examination. Unfortunately, Cohnheim neither shared Virchow's influence nor went to the trouble of clearly publishing his observations, and thus his contributions went largely unnoticed.

Later (1891), at the recently established Johns Hopkins Hospital and Medical School in Baltimore, William Welch used a carbon dioxide–freezing microtome to examine breast tissue removed by the preeminent surgeon William Halstead. Unfortunately, Welch did not appreciate the potential benefit of interpreting the frozen section slides immediately and so by the time he was ready to communicate the results, Halstead had already finished operating.

Welch's student Thomas S. Cullen is generally given credit for first publishing the technique for intraoperative frozen section in 1895. Cullen understood the principles of freezing and he sliced sections from intraoperative specimens by pre-fixing tissues in formalin.[4,5] Soon, the Mayo Clinic in Rochester, Illinois, led the way in refining the technique and a 1905 paper by Mayo's Louis B. Wilson provided a comprehensive description of the technique still used today. Though the paper has been criticized for not referencing the previous works of Cullen and others, the descriptions are clear, concise, and introduced many readers to the technique.[6-8] William Mayo reportedly encouraged the innovation and apparently often complained, "I wish you pathologists would find a way to tell us surgeons whether a growth is cancer or not while the patient is still on the table."

Key to the development of intraoperative tissue analysis is the manipulation of fresh tissue so that it is firmed and can be cut into thin (4-8 micron) sections for microscopic examination. A variety of methods had been used to firm the tissue in the early days: a hypertonic saline solution, heating techniques, and the topical application of zinc chloride.[9] Freezing the tissue became the method of choice as it offered a cheap and rapid way of hardening the tissue. Perhaps most importantly, freezing the tissue caused less disruption to the microscopic morphology, thereby allowing for a more accurate assessment. In the early days, innovative pathologists in colder climes left specimens outside to freeze. Modernization occurred in 1959 with the invention of the cryostat which allowed the rapid and consistent freezing of specimens. To assist the procedure, liquids were developed which allowed the tissue to both reach optimal cutting temperature and adhere to a metal plate. The aqueous solution of polyvinyl alcohol and polyethylene glycol became the most commonly used for sectioning in the cryostat.[10]

FROZEN SECTION PATHOLOGY BECOMES WIDELY USED

Frozen section diagnosis became an invaluable tool in assisting surgeons intraoperatively. Driving this advancement were the large and complex surgical procedures which became routine thanks to some remarkable innovations in anesthesiology and surgery. In the beginning, surgeons read the frozen section slides of tumors they had removed. It soon became obvious and accepted that the knowledge of a trained pathologist was essential.

The applications for frozen section assessments have expanded ever since its invention. Modern pathology laboratories routinely process specimens for intraoperative diagnosis and margin assessment of pulmonary, breast, soft tissue, genitourinary, gastrointestinal, head and neck, and nervous system resections.

INTRAOPERATIVE MARGIN ASSESSMENT IN CUTANEOUS SURGERY

The innovation of using intraoperative margin assessment for skin surgery is largely attributed to Frederic E. Mohs (1910-2002), a general surgeon based at the University of Wisconsin–Madison. Perhaps fortuitously (or if we are to give him more credit, probably wittingly), Mohs had spent time in a basic laboratory testing several chemical fixatives applied *in vivo* for animal studies. While evaluating a series of these "intralesional anticancer agents" on mice, Mohs (with his colleague, Michael Guyer) injected a solution of $ZnCl_2$ into murine skin tumors and found that it *not only* killed the cancer *but also* preserved the tissue structure. Thus, $ZnCl_2$ essentially served as a fixative, which gave Mohs the idea to use it to fix human skin cancers *in vivo*. The original paste contained $ZnCl_2$; a caustic extract and agglutinant, Sanguinaria canadensis root; and the inert permeant, stibnite. He made several modifications to the paste to improve its penetration and coagulability.[11,12] Following fixation, he excised the tumor and examined the margin histologically. Positive margins were mapped and further excised until clear margins were achieved. In 1941, Mohs reported his findings in the American Medical Association's Archives of Surgery. Mohs called this method and its preservative effect the "fixed-tissue" method of chemosurgery.[13,14]

At the time, fixation of the tissue *in vivo* was considered key as there was a perceived danger that the manipulation of fresh tissue through biopsy or partial excision could lead to the devastating consequence of dissemination of the malignancy. Due to the difficulty of applying the paste to structures around the eye—in what may be considered another stroke of fortune—Mohs used a frozen section as performed by pathologists at the time. Instead of using $ZnCl_2$ as a fixative, he simply anesthetized the area, excised the tumor, and moved directly to tissue preparation and histologic examination. He called this the "fresh tissue" method. After learning of the technique and being excited by the possibilities, dermatologic surgeon Theodore Tromovitch in 1963 began using the fresh-tissue technique on more and more body sites.[15,16] In December 1970 at the annual Chemosurgery Conference, he and Sam Stegman presented 104 cases of skin cancer surgery "without using zinc chloride chemical fixative," with only four recurrences. Subsequent papers reported high cure rates using the new form of chemosurgery, for example, an eight-year retrospective study reported a 97.2% cure rate for 532 lesions.[16]

One of the critical aspects of the Mohs technique is the way in which the tissue is manipulated so that the entire margin of the excision can be examined microscopically *en face,* that is, seen front on. Due to the difficulty in freezing the entire specimen (especially larger excisions with large amounts of adipose tissue which are more difficult to freeze), few pathologists at the time attempted complete margin assessment on skin excisions. The *in vivo* fixation caused the tissue to be hardened and ensured sectioning was much easier to deal with than fresh tissue. *En face* sectioning of the entire surgical margin was not invented with the Mohs technique, but it did popularize it.

AN ENTIRE FIELD IS BORN

Using frozen sections to assess the margins of an excision became known as margin control surgery (MCS). In the United States and then other countries, "Mohs micrographic surgery" became what many consider a distinct procedure within the MCS field, performed mainly by dermatologists who are usually involved in every aspect of the procedure: excision, histopathologic examination, and reconstruction. Training programs and accreditation helped standardize the technique and improved consistency and quality. In 1983, the first fellowship program was formally approved by the American College of Mohs Micrographic Surgery and Cutaneous Oncology (ACMMSCO). There are now numerous programs and approved fellowships in Australia, New Zealand, and Canada as well as other regulatory bodies supporting training and quality control in the procedure.

Given the challenges in processing skin specimens for frozen sections, the Mohs technique places particular emphasis on the competence and training of histotechnologists. This training was initially based on apprenticeships and on-the-job training. That changed in 1994 when the American Society for Mohs Histotechnology was formed, and the first Annual Meeting was held in 1995. Equivalent bodies continue to evolve in other countries, which helps to standardize quality, facilitates training, and encourages innovation.[17]

Of course, most patients worldwide have not had the benefit of access to Dr. Mohs or to those trained in his techniques. Frozen section examination of skin excisions performed outside the Mohs community, principally by pathologists, has remained somewhat less consistent with a wide range of techniques being deployed to examine specimens, ranging from "bread loafing" the specimen to sectioning exactly as was described by Dr. Mohs' fresh tissue technique. Increased emphasis on tissue sparing and reconstructive surgery has increased demand, with surgeons understanding its usefulness in intraoperative margin assessment before undertaking an immediate reconstruction.

In the early years, Mohs and his colleagues were principally using their technique on basal cell carcinoma (BCC) and squamous cell carcinoma (SCC). Surgical pathologists had gained experience diagnosing hundreds of distinct malignancies with frozen sections so it was a natural progression for MCS to become a popular technique for other cutaneous malignancies. Through the years, the literature has increasingly reported the utility of MCS in the management of cutaneous sarcomas, adnexal carcinomas, melanoma, and Merkel cell carcinoma.

Cutaneous MCS has benefited from the more general advancements in anatomic pathology. The application of immunohistochemistry in assessing frozen sections aids some practitioners in cases where a routine examination is more challenging, such as in melanoma. Telepathology has more recently emerged as a way of allowing specialist consultations in real time for difficult cases and its development has only increased with the rapid evolution of technologies, their affordability, and the general increase in acceptance, a state of affairs which was catalyzed by the COVID-19 pandemic.[18]

The term "slow Mohs" surgery has also gained popularity. In this procedure, the specimen is fixed in formalin, embedded in paraffin, and then manipulated in a manner to allow *en face* examination of the entire margin. This is useful in situations where an appropriate frozen section facility is not available or where frozen section interpretation is deemed too difficult. The wound is generally left open while the specimen is processed and the margins examined, and the patient returns at a later date for further excision of positive margin or reconstruction. Interestingly, in this context, the only aspect of Mohs' original technique which is applied to "slow Mohs" is the manipulation of the specimen to allow *en face* sectioning and examination of the entire margin. No *in vivo* fixative is used, and the processing and interpretation of the specimen is usually performed at an outside laboratory.

Novel ways of assessing margins have mirrored discoveries in medicine and science. Detection of cytogenetic aberrations in cancer led to technologies that attempt to rapidly assess the presence of tumor at margins intraoperatively.[19] Advancements in imaging technologies (e.g., reflectance confocal microscopy) and artificial intelligence offer promising methods of assessing margins *in vivo*. Despite these advancements, the use of histopathology remains the gold standard in margin assessment.

FINAL THOUGHTS

When considering the history, it should be remembered that hindsight tends to tell a different story when compared with what happened at the time. Decades of trial and error, dead ends, and serendipitous discoveries by prominent and obscure figures can be shaped into a tidy narrative and neatly summarized in a few paragraphs. Yet progress is never as straightforward as the history books present it. And now here we are, with journals and societies dedicated to a technique which, with the refinement of just a few subtle modifications, would still be recognizable to both "The Pope" Rudolf Virchow and Frederic Mohs.

References

1. Gal AA. In search of the origins of modern surgical pathology. *Adv Anat Pathol*. 2001;8(1):1-13.
2. Bracegirdle B. *A History of Microtechnique*. Ithaca, NY: Cornell University Press; 1978.
3. Lechago J. The frozen section: pathology in the trenches. *Arch Pathol Lab Med*. 2005;129(12):1529-1531.
4. Gal AA. In search of the origins of modern surgical pathology. *Adv Anat Pathol*. 2001;8:1-13.
5. Wright JR Jr. The development of the frozen section technique: the evolution of surgical biopsy, and the origins of surgical pathology. *Bull Hist Med*. 1985;59:295-326.
6. Bloodgood JC. Biopsy in diagnosis of malignancy. *South Med J*. 1927;20:18-28.
7. Gal AA. The centennial anniversary of the frozen section technique at the Mayo Clinic. *Arch Pathol Lab Med*. 2005;129(12):1532-1535.
8. Wilson LB. A method for the rapid preparation of fresh tissues for the microscope. *JAMA*. 1905;45:1737.
9. Goss GR. Frozen section: the stat test of clinical pathology? *Adv Med Lab*. 2001;13:8-12, 82.
10. Thomas VD, Aung PP, Rapini RP. Dermatopathology. In: Borczuk AC, Yantiss RK, Robinson BD, Scognamiglio T, D'Alfonso TM, eds. *Frozen Section Pathology*. Cham, Switzerland: Springer; 2021.
11. Swanson NA, Taylor WB. Plantar verrucous carcinoma. Literature review and treatment by the Mohs' chemosurgery technique. *Arch Dermatol*. 1980;116(7):794-797.
12. Shriner DL, McCoy DK, Goldberg DJ, Wagner RF. Mohs micrographic surgery. *J Am Acad Dermatol*. 1998;39(1):79-97.
13. Mohs FE, Chemosurgery A. Microscopically controlled method of cancer excision. *Arch Surg*. 1941;42(2):279-295.
14. Mohs FE. Chemosurgical treatment of cancer of the face; a microscopically controlled method of excision. *Arch Derm Syphilol*. 1947;56(2):143-156.
15. Brodland DG, Amonette R, Hanke CW, Robins P. The history and evaluation of Mohs micrographic surgery. *Dermatol Surg*. 2000;26:303-307.
16. Tromovitch TA, Stegman SJ. Microscopic-controlled excision of cutaneous tumors: chemosurgery, fresh tissue technique. *Cancer*. 1978;41:653-658.
17. McLeod MP, Choudhary S, Nouri K. An introduction to mohs micrographic surgery. In: Nouri K, ed. *Mohs Micrographic Surgery*. London: Springer; 2012.
18. Emanuel PO, Patel R, Zwi J, Cheng D, Izzard M. Utility of teledermatopathology for intraoperative margin assessment of melanoma in situ, lentigo maligna type: a 6 year community practice experience. *Eur J Surg Oncol*. 2021;47(5):1140-1144.
19. Jaiswal YP, Gadkari RU. Evaluation of role of intraoperative cytology technique in diagnosis and management of cancer. *J Cytol*. 2020;37(3):126-130.

2

Multidisciplinary Approach

Patrick Emanuel / Rajan S. Patel

Intraoperative MCS Outside of the MMS Setting
    MDMs
    Telepathology
    Slow Mohs
Summary

Distinct from other cancers, most skin cancers are managed in a doctor's office or ambulatory clinic in the community rather than in a referral hospital. For this reason, skin cancer patients can navigate the health system without the input of the integrated team approach which may otherwise be needed. As is the case with practically all aspects of medicine, both communication between specialists and integration of care are key components in reaching the best patient outcomes.

INTRAOPERATIVE MCS OUTSIDE OF THE MMS SETTING

To assess surgical margins intraoperatively, the broad range of medical specialists involved in skin cancer surgery typically rely on their local pathologists who are also involved in the processing of the specialists' regular specimens. The laboratory may be within an operating room suite or at a separate location, in which case communication between the laboratory and the surgeon is important while the tumor is being removed, orientated, labeled, and transported.

To facilitate communication, photographs of the tumor before excision and of the specimen with orientation can easily be sent to the pathologist. Teleconference programs can also be used so that the pathologist is able to see the tumor before it is excised and discuss orientation and clinical details with the surgeon intraoperatively. A workflow of the process is summarized in **Table 2.1**.

Many surgeons are unaware of the method pathologists use to assess margins. And if the services within a laboratory are delegated by the pathologist to another staff member such as a technician, the pathologist may also be unaware of exactly what takes place in the examination of a specimen. It is important that the surgeon has a good understanding of the procedures involved in order to provide the most appropriate specimen and information required for accurate margin assessment. For example, sending piecemeal biopsies of the peripheral margins may seem like an attractive idea to the surgeon but these can

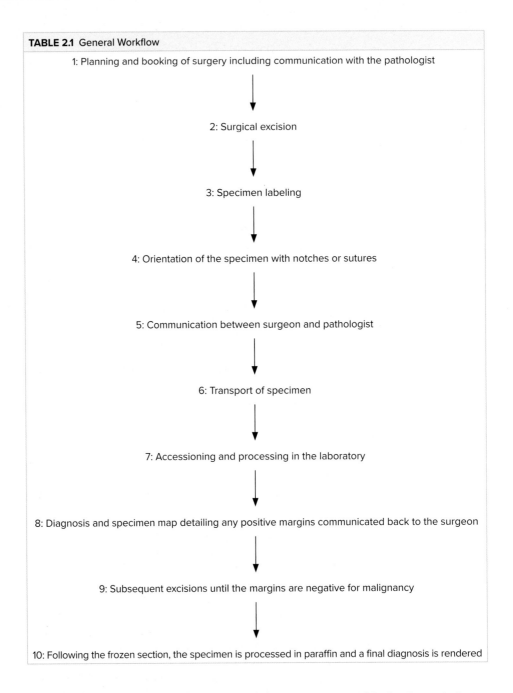

TABLE 2.1 General Workflow

1: Planning and booking of surgery including communication with the pathologist

2: Surgical excision

3: Specimen labeling

4: Orientation of the specimen with notches or sutures

5: Communication between surgeon and pathologist

6: Transport of specimen

7: Accessioning and processing in the laboratory

8: Diagnosis and specimen map detailing any positive margins communicated back to the surgeon

9: Subsequent excisions until the margins are negative for malignancy

10: Following the frozen section, the specimen is processed in paraffin and a final diagnosis is rendered

make a subsequent complete assessment of the margin impossible for the pathologist. Thick, wide excisions for small tumors can cause processing difficulty and delays. It is essential that the surgeon appreciate that precise technical expertise and time are required to complete a full-margin assessment.

A key difference between this multidisciplinary approach and Mohs micrographic surgery (MMS) is that, in MMS, the physician performing the excision usually also interprets the pathology. This allows an opportunity for clinicopathologic correlation which is widely accepted as one of the reasons MMS has been so successful as a procedure. Clinicopathologic correlation is an invaluable tool for anyone practicing dermatopathology (some rashes are practically impossible to distinguish histologically without assessing how the rash is manifesting clinically). However, the significance of clinical correlation is less well described in the context of margin control surgery (MCS). And less attention has been paid to the potential for bias being introduced when a surgeon also interprets the pathology.

Prospect theory is a Nobel prize-winning economic construct which proposes that logical assumptions are not always represented in actual choices, largely because logical assumptions do not consider cognitive biases. What cognitive biases may exist if a physician performing an excision also interprets the pathology slides? Biases arise from a wide range of factors such as the interaction with the patient (e.g., is this patient likely to sue me?), knowledge of the patient's insurance, or time pressures from a full operating list. In these scenarios, can we be sure that the operating surgeon is not biased to some degree about what they are interpreting down the microscope? Is a difficult patient more likely to have an unusual hair follicle interpreted as a possible basal cell carcinoma (BCC) and therefore have an extra level removed? This is not to say that these biases necessarily outweigh the insight gleaned from clinicopathologic correlation when the surgeon interprets their own pathology, but at the very least these need to be considered by the surgeon who is operating in this environment. The factors distinguishing the multidisciplinary approach from MMS are summarized in **Table 2.2**.

MDMs

Multidisciplinary meetings (MDMs) are a cornerstone of treatment at leading cancer centers and are commonplace in larger centers treating skin cancers. In fact, an MDM is required for accreditation by the American College of Surgeons' Commission on Cancer. In other territories such as the United Kingdom and Australasia, MDMs are an essential component of the national standard for cancer care.[1] In many places, doctors practicing in the community have a regional MDM to which they can refer patients and/or attend themselves.

TABLE 2.2 Compared with MMS
Advantages: • Viable option in locations not served by Mohs surgeons   • More complicated, larger surgical excisions (e.g., with involvement of deep structures) performed by specialist surgeons can be examined   • Access to specialist dermatopathologist or anatomic pathologists in cases where unusual tumors are excised   • Direct correlation between frozen section findings and subsequent permanent sections which may be performed in the same laboratory   • Decreased cognitive bias (see discussion of prospect theory)
Disadvantages: • Less clinicopathologic correlation   • More steps in procedure means higher chance of error   • Less correlation/ability to judge orientation of positive margins and extent of surgery for subsequent levels   • Less uniformity in processing techniques

In addition to surgeons, dermatologists, and pathologists, the skin cancer MDMs are attended by a team which commonly includes general practitioners, radiation and medical oncologists, radiologists, nurses, and other allied health professionals. In these meetings, any aspect of the care of the patient may be discussed, including the use of MCS.

Deciding which patients with skin cancer should be submitted to these MDMs can be challenging. Usually, high-risk cases are considered, but how these are defined is subject to geographic variation, and criteria are tailored to the community need (see example in **Table 2.3**). It is in some ways a balancing act between capturing all the patients who would benefit from the opinions of various specialist groups and how many cases can practically be reviewed by a given MDM. For example, if the outdated American Joint Committee on Cancer (AJCC) (7th edition) staging protocol were to be used as an entrance requirement, the MDM could soon become overwhelmed as many more cancers were once considered high-risk. Many centers in the United States rely on the criteria set out by the National Comprehensive Cancer Network (NCCN). The NCCN recommends multidisciplinary consultation specifically for problematic tumors such as those with nerve involvement or positive surgical margins.

In addition to the discussion of surgical and pathologic considerations, a discussion of adjuvant radiation, chemotherapy, and patient follow-up is common. A survey of the utility of these meetings showed various aspects of the meetings are deemed valuable by almost all attendees (**Table 2.4**).

In the context of MCS, these meetings may serve as an opportunity to review the pathology of a biopsy and discuss specific issues related to the specimen, for example, the need to examine lymph nodes or larger nerves intraoperatively.[3] Discussion may include the necessity of using a general anesthetic and whether intraoperative margin assessment is feasible given the time restraints. The pathology review may discover that the tumor would be very difficult to see with frozen section examination and that paraffin processing is more appropriate (slow Mohs).

As reported in the literature, patients discussed at MDMs may receive a change in diagnosis (18.4%-29%) or treatment plan (20%-52%).[3,4] A review of the histopathology may be

---

TABLE 2.3 Example of Criteria for Inclusion into MDM[2]

- All patients with high-risk squamous cell carcinoma (SCC) and BCC involving excision margins or are recurrent
- Skin cancers in patients who are immunocompromised or those with genetic predisposition
- Patients with metastatic SCC or BCC diagnosed at presentation or on follow-up
- Patients who may benefit from radiotherapy or chemotherapy
- Patients who may be eligible for entry into clinical trials
- Specific challenging management issues such as cognitive impairment or medical comorbidities

---

TABLE 2.4 Utility of MDM Conference[3]

- Enhanced communication among physicians
- Continuing medical education for physicians
- Encourages use of most recent guidelines for management
- More treatment options for patients
- Opportunity for physicians, nurses, allied health professionals to discuss cases together

Reproduced with permission from Mori S, Navarrete-Dechent C, Petukhova TA, et al. Tumor Board Conferences for multidisciplinary skin cancer management: a survey of US Cancer Centers. J Natl Compr Canc Netw. 2018;16(10):1209-1215.

an opportunity to suggest additional testing, for example, additional molecular or immunohistochemical markers for diagnosis or therapy. Frequently, more clinical details come to light which help the pathologist formulate the final diagnosis such as previous pathology results, the possibility of a cutaneous metastasis from another site, and known comorbid diseases.

Telepathology

Telepathology facilitates the collaboration between surgeons and pathologists as well as among specialist pathologists. Advances in technology have enabled remote reporting of dermatopathology using whole slide imaging (WSI) and real-time video streaming. With WSI systems, instead of a microscope, pathologists use their computers to view slides scanned at a different site (**Fig. 2.1**). Various regulatory bodies have been involved in the approval of telepathology internationally. A breakthrough in the acceptance of slide scanning came with the approval of specific systems by the US Food and Drug Administration for diagnostic purposes.[5,6]

There is a wide range of WSI options. The best systems currently available have high-end digital camera sensors, sophisticated computer software, and call for a high internet bandwidth. Unsurprisingly, these systems are expensive. However, the prices of these devices are set to reduce, as is the time required to scan individual slides. WSI is therefore likely to play a more integral role in the future. In the MCS sphere, there is currently a range of more feasible options. Dynamic systems with real-time consultation with a video stream are very useful. In this arrangement, the pathologist usually drives the microscope

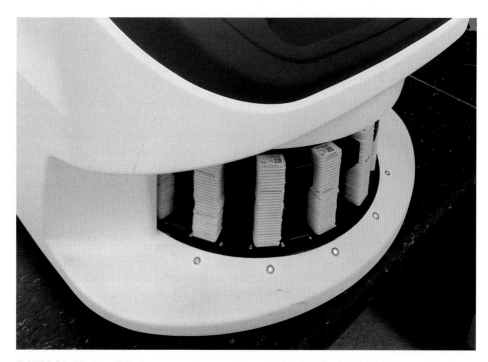

FIGURE 2.1. **Modern slide scanners can scan a large volume of slides and have become an integral part of some pathology laboratories.** Scanned images of the slides are stored on a server for the pathologist to view remotely.

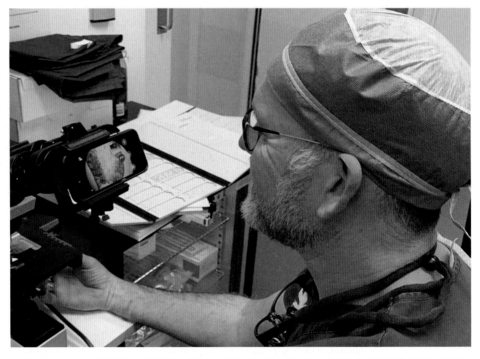

FIGURE 2.2. **A smartphone is attached to the microscope with an adapter.** A teleconference application allows the pathologist to review the slide remotely together with the surgeon. The case can be discussed while examining the slides, functioning much like a multiheaded microscope.

remotely with a robotic stage and views the video stream captured on an attached camera. Instead of using a robot, an alternative is for the surgeon to drive the slide around the microscope stage manually so that the pathologist at a remote location and the surgeon view the same slide together. This serves much like a multiheaded microscope; the surgeon and the pathologist can discuss the case in real time, closely examine areas of interest, and/or assess entire margins. A range of devices has been used since around 2000. Given the astonishing advancement in the quality of smartphone images and videoconference applications (e.g., Facetime, WhatsApp, Zoom), remote consultation with a telephone is a possibility and is gaining popularity (**Fig. 2.2**).[6,7]

Telepathology during MCS can facilitate intraoperative case consultation with a specialist dermatopathologist. This can be particularly helpful in difficult cases such as the interpretation of the margins of melanoma or incidental findings such as lymphoma or a possible second carcinoma (**Fig. 2.3**).

The COVID-19 pandemic catalyzed the adoption of telepathology in routine practice. In the United States, Clinical Laboratory Improvement Amendments (CLIA) dictates that pathologists must practice in a CLIA-approved workplace. Due to the transmission risk of COVID-19 associated with busy workplaces, regulators in the United States temporarily waived this requirement so that pathologists could work at non-CLIA-approved sites (i.e., the pathologists' home). Similar moves occurred internationally. In many cases, the telepathology systems had been previously validated but the need to keep pathology services functioning during these difficult times increased their adoption.

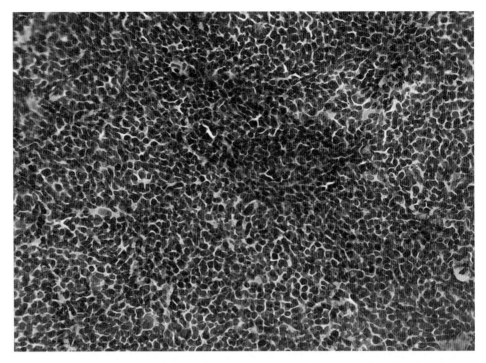

FIGURE 2.3. **This is a tumor viewed remotely via telepathology.** It was encountered incidentally during the excision of a BCC. The operating surgeon was unsure whether this was an undifferentiated carcinoma. The consulting pathologist concluded it was likely a lymphoma. No further excision was performed and tissue was sent fresh for flow cytometry and in formalin to the laboratory. The final diagnosis was mantle cell lymphoma diagnosed as a result of MCS.

Slow Mohs

In slow Mohs surgery, the specimen is fixed in formalin, embedded in paraffin, and then manipulated in a manner to allow *en face* examination of the entire margin. The specimen is usually processed rapidly (often overnight), and positive margins are mapped. The patient returns to the surgeon when the pathology has been examined. If the margins are clear, reconstruction is performed in the second surgical session. If the margins are positive, further tissue is removed from the involved area and the process is repeated until the tumor is clear. Though this process has been used for many decades without much attention outside of the pathology community, it gained popularity in the dermatology community when it was first described formally by Breuninger et al. in 1988[8] and became known as slow Mohs. It is a useful method when an appropriate frozen section facility is not available or in cases where frozen section interpretation is considered too difficult. Given that the specimen is processed in paraffin, interpretation of the morphology is easier for the pathologist. The pathologist can also rely on immunohistochemical studies which are readily available in a pathology laboratory but are not widely used in the frozen section context.

Interestingly, the only aspect of Mohs' original technique which is applied to slow Mohs is the manipulation of the specimen to allow *en face* sectioning and examination of the entire margin to provide mapping of the tumor. No *in vivo* fixative is used and the processing and interpretation of the specimen are usually performed at an outside laboratory by a pathologist. Key points relevant to the slow Mohs technique are summarized in **Table 2.5.**

TABLE 2.5 Slow Mohs Technique

Advantages:
- Specimens are processed in paraffin, so interpretation is generally easier than with frozen section slides.
- Immunohistochemistry can be readily performed.
- Manipulation and cutting of the specimen are easier.

Disadvantages:
- Time-consuming and generally takes 24-48 hours for each margin assessment to be completed in the laboratory.
- The wound is usually left open, increasing the risk of infection. If the wound is left open for a protracted period, granulation and distortion of the corresponding margins is a risk.
- The patient needs to return for various sessions over many days if the margins are positive.

SUMMARY

Multidisciplinary MCS usually involves the operating surgeon working together with a pathologist. Close communication is key to the success of this arrangement. The collegial approach encouraged through MDMs results in good outcomes for patients. The role of telepathology is expanding and it can be used intraoperatively to allow real-time consultations.

References

1. Department of Health. *Manual for Cancer Services.* London: Department of Health; 2011.
2. Newlands C, Currie R, Memon A, Whitaker S, Woolford T. Non-melanoma skin cancer: United Kingdom National Multidisciplinary Guidelines. *J Laryngol Otol.* 2016;130(S2): S125-S132.
3. Mori S, Navarrete-Dechent C, Petukhova TA, et al. Tumor Board Conferences for Multidisciplinary Skin Cancer Management: a survey of us cancer centers. *J Natl Compr Canc Netw.* 2018;16(10):1209-1215.
4. Basta YL, Bolle S, Fockens P, Tytgat KMAJ. The value of multidisciplinary team meetings for patients with gastrointestinal malignancies: a systematic review. *Annals of Surgical Oncology.* 2017;24:2669-2678.
5. Evans AJ, Bauer TW, Bui MM, et al. US Food and Drug Administration approval of whole slide imaging for primary diagnosis: a key milestone is reached and new questions are raised. *Arch Pathol Lab Med.* 2018;142(11):1383-1387.
6. Laggis CW, Bailey EE, Novoa R, et al. Validation of image quality and diagnostic accuracy using a mobile phone camera microscope adaptor compared with glass slide review in teledermatopathology. *Am J Dermatopathol.* 2020;42(5):349-353.
7. Emanuel PO, Patel R, Zwi J, Cheng D, Izzard M. Utility of teledermatopathology for intraoperative margin assessment of melanoma in situ, lentigo maligna type: a 6-year community practice experience. *Eur J Surg Oncol.* 2021;47(5):1140-1144.
8. Breuninger H, Schaumburg-Lever G. Control of excisional margins by conventional histopathological techniques in the treatment of skin tumours. An alternative to Mohs' technique. *J Pathol.* 1988;154:167-171.

3

Mohs Micrographic Surgery

Rebecca Kleinerman / Patrick Emanuel

Definition
Indications for MMS
Why Recommend MMS?
    Efficacy
    Tissue Preservation
Practical Issues

The Surgical Procedure
Specimen Preparation
Reconstruction
Training Surgeons and Technicians
Cost-Effectiveness
Summary

Few medical procedures have the mystique that surrounds Mohs micrographic surgery (MMS). While most physicians whose work involves treating skin cancer understand it in principle, many are less aware of what is wholly involved or how it is performed. Some patients may have also heard of it and, after conducting a little research, concluded that it is what they want for their skin cancer as the term is practically synonymous with the highest chance of cure. They can view MMS as a silver bullet, a mysterious yet infallible solution to their condition; one minor procedure and, like magic, their lesion will be fixed. While there is a reason for this optimism, the physician must rely on deeper knowledge and careful judgment.

MMS has enjoyed enormous success as a procedure, probably more so than any other form of margin control surgery (MCS). Training programs and quality assurance programs help ensure standardization and quality. Societies with annual meetings encourage collegiality and innovation. Specialist technicians have also developed societies, training programs, and continued education. With these developments, its popularity has increased around the world and its use has diversified to treat an ever-wider range of tumors and clinical situations.

DEFINITION

There seems to be a variety of definitions for what MMS is. It has been defined as a procedure performed by a dermatologist who acts as both the surgeon and pathologist. The dermatologist performs the surgery to remove the tumor, examines the margins intraoperatively with horizontal frozen sections, maps positive margins and re-excises the positive areas until the margins are clear, and then typically performs the reconstruction. But there is considerable variability internationally. For example, sometimes the surgeon is not a dermatologist, sometimes a pathologist is involved in interpreting the slides, sometimes the reconstruction is performed by a reconstructive surgeon, and sometimes the Mohs surgeon is only involved in the interpretation of the histopathology slides. The term has been stretched further still: Some apply this term to any procedure which involves examination of 100% of the margins intraoperatively regardless of the pathology processing used or the specialists involved. Further confusion is added by the use of the term "slow Mohs," which usually means examination of the entire margin with formalin-fixed paraffin-embedding processing.

INDICATIONS FOR MMS

The suitability for MMS was formalized in the United States with the appropriate use criteria (AUC) publication produced in 2012 by the American Academy of Dermatology (AAD) in collaboration with the American College of Mohs Surgery, the American Society for Dermatologic Surgery, and the American Society for Mohs Surgery. Clinical scenarios were developed following consultation with 70 experts and then a panel of raters scored the appropriateness of MMS for each scenario. The panel consisted of 17 dermatologists, of which eight were practicing MMS surgeons. Similar guidelines have been developed by equivalent bodies in other countries and territories.

The AAD has an app (https://www.aad.org/member/publications/apps/mohs) that helpfully provides support on the appropriateness of MMS for 270 distinct scenarios.

The resultant AUC for the appropriateness of MMS are divided into three anatomic sites: High, medium, and low risk.[1,2]

Area with high risk, Area H: "Mask areas" of face (central face, eyelids [including inner/outer canthi], eyebrows, nose, lips [cutaneous/mucosal/vermillion], chin, ear and periauricular skin/sulci, temple), genitalia (including perineal and perianal), hands, feet, nail units, ankles, and nipples/areola.

In this area, MMS was considered always appropriate for basal cell carcinoma (BCC), squamous cell carcinoma (SCC), and melanoma in situ (MIS). MMS was not considered appropriate for Actinic keratosis (AK) (**Fig. 3.1**).

Area with medium risk, Area M: Cheeks, forehead, scalp, neck, jawline, and pretibial surface.

In this area, MMS was considered always appropriate for BCC, SCC, and MIS except for small superficial BCCs (0.5 cm and less). AK is also considered inappropriate.

Area with low risk, Area L: Trunk and extremities (excluding pretibial surface, hands, feet, nail units, and ankles).

In this area, the appropriateness is a little more complicated and is summarized in **Table 3.1**. It should be noted that superficial BCC is never considered appropriate for MMS in low-risk areas.

MMS was also deemed appropriate for a wide range of rarer tumors including adenoid cystic carcinoma, adnexal carcinoma, apocrine/eccrine carcinoma, atypical fibroxanthoma, dermatofibrosarcoma protuberans, extramammary Paget disease, leiomyosarcoma, microcystic adnexal carcinoma (sclerosing sweat duct carcinoma), mucinous carcinoma, and sebaceous carcinoma in all locations. Angiosarcoma was deemed uncertain.

MMS for Merkel cell carcinoma was determined to be appropriate in areas H and M. The AUC for MCC were determined by considering MMS as monotherapy, while the possibility of adjuvant radiation therapy was not factored into the final AUC decision.

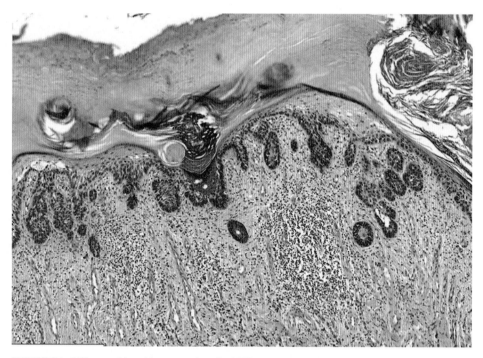

FIGURE 3.1. **AK is considered inappropriate for MMS.** A degree of subjectivity does come in to diagnosing AK. The example shown here of proliferative AK may be considered a superficially invasive squamous cell carcinoma by some dermatopathologists.

WHY RECOMMEND MMS?

Central to this technique is the high cure rates and the ability to preserve normal tissue in cosmetically sensitive areas. The recommendation for MMS treatment should be made after careful evaluation not only of the histology and location of the tumor but also of the patient's characteristics. MMS may at times be a long procedure and some patients find it difficult to cope. Specific care should be taken with patients with dementia, severe arthritis, or poor sphincter control.

Efficacy

MMS has consistently shown excellent efficacy rates. In a large cohort, the five-year recurrence rates for primary BCCs were 8.7% for non-MMS and 1% for MMS. The figures for recurrent tumors were 19.9% and 5.6%, respectively. Others quote recurrence rates for primary BCCs treated with wide local excision (WLE) versus MMS as 10% and 1%, respectively. Five-year recurrence rates for recurrent BCCs with WLE are 5% to 40% compared with those treated with MMS, which are 3% to 8%.[3]

For SCCs smaller than 2 cm in diameter, a five-year cure rate of 99% with MMS has been quoted. Tumors between 2 cm and 3 cm in diameter have an 82% five-year cure rate, whereas tumors larger than 3 cm have a 59% cure rate.[4]

Rowe et al. also studied prognostic factors for local recurrence, metastasis, and survival rate in SCC of the skin, ear, and lip by reviewing studies conducted between 1940 and 1992. Their findings are summarized in **Table 3.2**.

TABLE 3.1 Appropriateness of MMS for Tumors in Area L (Low Risk)[1,2]

Area L	Always Appropriate	Uncertain	Not Appropriate
BCC	Primary: - Aggressive ≥ 0.6 cm - Nodular > 2 cm - Nodular (IC) ≥ 1.1 cm Recurrent: - Aggressive - Nodular	Primary: - Aggressive ≤ 0.5 cm - Nodular 1.1-2 cm - Nodular (IC) 0.6-1 cm - Superficial (IC) ≥ 1.1 cm	Primary: - Nodular ≤ 1 cm - Nodular (IC) ≤ 0.5 cm - Superficial - Superficial (IC) ≤ 1 cm Recurrent: - Superficial
SCC	Primary or recurrent: - Aggressive Primary > 2 cm: - Nonaggressive - SCC in situ Primary ≥ 1.1 cm: - Nonaggressive (IC) - KA-type SCC - SCC in situ (IC) Recurrent: - KA-type SCC - Nonaggressive - KA-type SCC (IC) ≥ 0.6 cm	Primary 1-2 cm: - Nonaggressive - SCC in situ Primary ≤ 1 cm: - Nonaggressive (IC) Primary 0.6-1 cm: - SCC in situ (IC) Primary ≤ 0.5 cm: - KA-type SCC (IC) Recurrent: - SCC in situ	Primary ≤ 0.5 cm: - SCC in situ (IC) Primary ≤ 1 cm: - Nonaggressive - KA-type SCC - SCC in situ Primary or recurrent: - AK with focal SCC in situ
MIS	Recurrent: LM, MIS	Primary: LM, MIS	

IC, immunocompromised.
For BCC, aggressive subtypes were defined as:
Morpheaform/fibrosing/sclerosing Infiltrating
Perineural invasion
Metatypical/keratotic Micronodular

For SCC, aggressive subtypes were defined as:
Sclerosing, basosquamous (excluding keratotic BCC), small cell, poorly or undifferentiated (characterized by a high degree of nuclear polymorphism, high mitotic rate, or low degree of keratinization) perineural/perivascular invasion, clear cell, lymphoepithelial, sarcomatoid, Breslow depth 2 mm or greater, Clark level IV or greater

TABLE 3.2 Recurrence Rates[5]

	MMS (%)	Non-MMS (%)
SCC of skin/lip	3	17
SCC of ear	5	19
Recurrent SCC	10	23
Perineural SCC	0	47
SCC > 2 cm	25	41
Poorly differentiated tumors	33	54

It should, however, be noted that much of the literature has compared MMS with WLE. It has even been suggested that the only way in which the entire margin can be examined is with MMS.[6] This is not necessarily the case. Pathologists are generally well-versed in various methods of processing specimens and there are various options for examining the entire margin histopathologically (see Chap. 6, Specimen Preparation). When this comparison with other techniques is made, WLE is probably interpreted as an excision of a tumor with the recommended surgical margins followed by a bread-loaf pathologic examination. Given this and many confounding variables, it is difficult, for example, to compare MMS with WLE with complete margin assessment performed in paraffin (with the use of immunohistochemistry in difficult cases). A criticism some have made against MMS is that no randomized control trials have been conducted to illustrate its effectiveness, but this is a near-impossible task.

Tissue Preservation

Bumsted et al. demonstrated that there was 180% excess tissue taken when BCCs smaller than 3 cm are excised with 8-mm margins using a WLE as compared with MMS. Downes showed that Mohs surgery preserved 41% more tissue than a traditional excision for periocular BCCs. This is a key factor in a positive cosmetic outcome.[7,8] As discussed in other parts of this book, tissue preservation is important, but operating to the anatomy is also a consideration. Specifically, excising a tumor with extremely narrow margins may seem ideal, but if the tumor crosses facial subunits then the tissue conservation may not be important.[9]

PRACTICAL ISSUES

MMS is usually performed in a dermatology office or ambulatory surgical center. Consistent with any surgical procedure, consideration needs to be given to antibiotic prophylaxis. In 2007, the American Heart Association's guidelines recommended the use of endocarditis prophylaxis only in cases involving infected skin or in patients with a range of medical issues such as a history of previous endocarditis, cardiac transplant, cardiac valve disease, and prosthetic implants. Generally, it is recommended that patients continue their anticoagulant medications during MMS, but for patients receiving warfarin, the coagulation studies should be checked a week before surgery and surgery should be avoided in patients with supratherapeutic anticoagulation.

Obtaining informed consent before MMS is somewhat involved when compared with other dermatologic procedures. The final defect size and subsequent repair are estimated before the procedure. There exists a high likelihood that the tumor may extend beyond what is evident to the naked eye, referred to as subclinical extension. The surgeon must explain to the patient that the visible part of the tumor is often the "tip of the iceberg," and the tumor may extend past what is clinically evident. Factors associated with subclinical extension include tumors greater than 1 cm in diameter, recurrent tumors, and tumors with fibrosis noted on initial biopsy. Given the possibility of larger defects than anticipated, it is essential to discuss expectations of final defect sizes and potential repair options with the patient.

Once informed consent is obtained, the biopsy site is identified. This is not always easy, especially for small lesions and biopsies taken months or years earlier. One study found that about 9% of patients could not identify their biopsy site at the time of surgery.[10] Finding the surgical site may be further complicated if the patient has had multiple lesions biopsied. The patient can sometimes help in the identification of the lesion, but it should be noted that it is not infrequent for the patient to be mistaken. There are various techniques for mitigating this risk, including cell phone photography ("selfies") at the time of biopsy and gauze dermabrasion to uncover the weakened tissue at the initial biopsy site.[11,12]

THE SURGICAL PROCEDURE

The area is cleansed with an antiseptic and a surgical ink pen is used to delineate clinically evident tumor or boundaries of the biopsy scar. The area is anesthetized with local anesthetic and then the tumor is usually curetted to debulk the tumor and allow for easier manipulation of the specimen. A line is then drawn around the defect (about 1-2 mm around it) and marks are either drawn or nicked (notched) with the scalpel for orientation (depending on the specimen, a single nick will be made at 12 o'clock or multiple nicks will be made at 12, 3, 6, and 9 o'clock). For the excision, the surgical blade is best oriented at a 45° angle to the skin, which is referred to as beveling, and is important in creating quality slides. A key part of the MMS technique is the removal: Careful attention is needed to excise a specimen with a flat, horizontal plane at the deep margin. This deep plane should be just beneath the curettage plane so that a thin disk with a flat base is removed. The specimen may be removed with a scalpel or with sharp scissors to create an even plane at the deep margin. Attention needs to be paid to where the orientation marks are once the specimen has been removed and placed on gauze.

SPECIMEN PREPARATION

In MMS, the specimen is excised with angulated radial margins (the bevel) and a flat deep margin to aid in the embedding (**Fig. 3.2**). Also see the chapter on specimen preparation.

The result of the processing is *en face* frozen sections of the entire margin (**Fig. 3.3**).

Any positive areas are mapped and these areas are re-excised until a negative surgical margin is achieved. Though this is usually quite a simple map, more extensive lesions require large complex maps (**Fig. 3.4**). Some surgeons prefer dividing the specimens into quadrants to assist in orientation. The pieces are processed separately, which is more time-consuming as more tissue blocks need to be processed.

RECONSTRUCTION

Following complete clearance of the tumor, the Mohs surgeon prepares for reconstruction of the surgical defect. Mohs surgeons use a variety of techniques when closing both simple and more complex skin defects, including second-intention healing, layered closures, skin flaps, and skin grafts. Deep wounds on the nose may require cartilage grafting as well. Anatomic location of the defect, depth of the wound, reservoir of nearby skin, and adjacent anatomic structures are all taken into consideration while planning the defect repair as this may affect function and aesthetics.

Delaying repair is an additional consideration for larger defects and may be required when more complicated reconstructions are necessary. Sometimes allowing wounds to granulate for a period, followed by a delayed flap or graft, may restore contour more adequately than immediate repair. There is considerable nuance to reconstruction that comes with training and experience.

TRAINING SURGEONS AND TECHNICIANS

There is a range of training arrangements internationally. In the United States, the Accreditation Council for Graduate Medical Education accredits training in fellowship training in Micrographic Surgery and Dermatologic Oncology. These are usually one year in length and encompass (among other things) all aspects of Mohs surgery including exposure to 500 cases with a range of complexity. A board examination in Micrographic Dermatologic Surgery was initiated in 2021 to standardize knowledge of the technique, and fellowship-trained Mohs surgeons as well as those practicing Mohs surgery in the United States were invited to sit for the examination within five years. Similarly, the British Society of Dermatologic Surgery and the Australasian College of Dermatologists offer

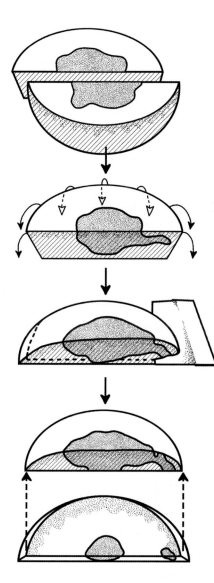

FIGURE 3.2. The specimen is manipulated so that the radial margins are in the same plane as the deep margin (curved arrows). With the entire radial and deep margin in the same plane, the histologic sections are cut horizontally, allowing microscopic examination of the entire margin. In this graphic, the tumor can be seen in the resulting section of the margin at the bottom.

training programs and credentialing to become an approved provider. Following completion of training, the continued education and review of practice are required for maintenance of certification.

Internationally, not all dermatologists who perform MMS are fellowship-trained. There are a variety of shorter courses available, and some learn through more informal apprenticeships. As with any skill, repeated practice, especially practice under supervision, increases expertise. There are many factors to consider and the ability to practice may depend on insurance companies and local regulations. The MMS laboratory is also subject to regulation. For example, in the United States, a Clinical Laboratory Improvement Amendments certificate and inspection are required. In many countries, a pathologist must interpret the MMS slides.

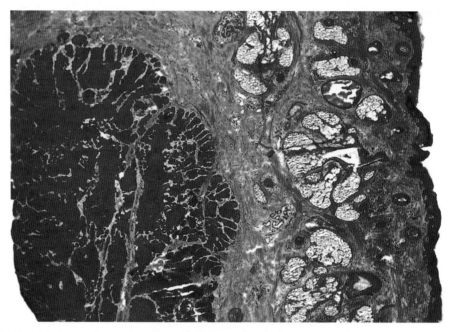

FIGURE 3.3. Photo of an *en face* frozen section with nodular BCC at the deep margin of the speci-men. An additional level of tissue needs to be taken and assessed for clearance.

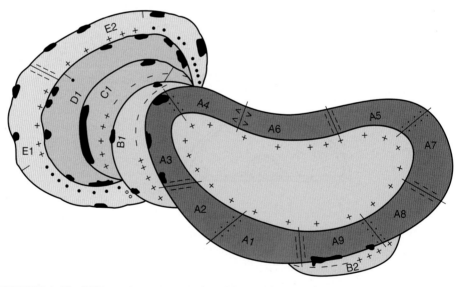

FIGURE 3.4. The MMS map is a representation of the excision with the positive margins drawn. Usually, this is a basic process, but it needs to be precise so the surgeon knows exactly where to re-excise on the patient. In more difficult cases, the map may be quite complicated as seen here.

The American Society for Mohs Histotechnology offers training programs to provide improved slide preparation technique and this society provides extremely useful opportu-nities for technicians to refine their skills. Internationally, most technicians have a back-ground in laboratory science and learn the specifics of MMS tissue processing "on the job."

COST-EFFECTIVENESS

It is difficult to generalize about the cost of MMS as this varies considerably in different countries and territories. In the United States, a 2012 study by Ravitskiy, Brodland, and Zitelli examined the costs of 406 consecutive cases in which MMS was compared with WLE. When factoring in surgical and laboratory fees, they concluded that MMS was less expensive than a WLE with permanent section analysis.[13] Excision in an ambulatory surgical facility with frozen section analysis done by a separate pathologist was considerably more expensive. European studies have demonstrated to a lesser degree the cost-effectiveness of MMS when compared with WLE.[14] In addition, a 2016 retrospective Iranian study demonstrated the cost-effectiveness of MMS compared with WLE.[15]

SUMMARY

MMS has a variety of definitions internationally but most of its basic principles are clear. Namely, the technique implies the excision of the specimen, examination of the entire margin intraoperatively, mapping of the positive margins, re-excision until the margins are clear, and finally reconstruction. It has become increasingly standardized in certain parts of the world due to the formation of professional societies, training programs, and AUC. These factors and the excellent cure rates suggest its continued success and continuing expansion of utility. Clinical photographs of a standard case are shown in **Fig. 3.5.**

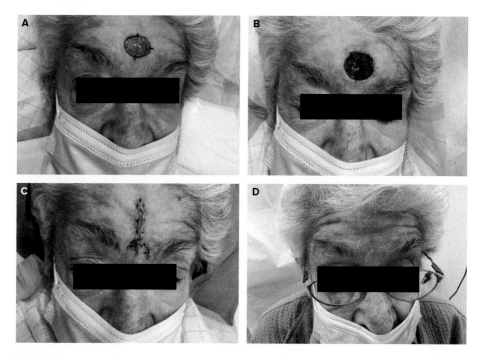

FIGURE 3.5. (A-D): A largish forehead BCC was excised with the MMS method. Note the three orienting nicks (notches) cut before excision (A). The tumor was excised with the surgical blade oriented at a 45° angle to the skin, which is referred to as beveling. Positive margins were excised until histologic clearance was achieved (B). Following histologic clearance, linear closure resulted in an excellent cosmetic result (C, D).

References

1. Ad Hoc Task Force, Connolly SM, Baker DR, et al. AAD/ACMS/ASDSA/ASMS 2012 appropriate use criteria for Mohs micrographic surgery: a report of the American Academy of Dermatology, American College of Mohs Surgery, American Society for Dermatologic Surgery Association, and the American Society for Mohs Surgery. *J Am Acad Dermatol.* 2012;67:531-550.

2. Blechman AB, Patterson JW, Russell MA. Application of Mohs micrographic surgery appropriate-use criteria to skin cancers at a university health system. *J Am Acad Dermatol.* 2014;71(1):29-35.

3. Rowe DE, Carroll RJ, Day CL Jr. Mohs surgery is the treatment of choice for recurrent (previously treated) basal cell carcinoma. *J Dermatol Surg Oncol.* 1989;15(4):424-431.

4. Marks R. Squamous cell carcinoma. *Lancet.* 1996;347(9003):735-738.

5. Rowe DE, Carroll RJ, Day CL Jr. Prognostic factors for local recurrence, metastasis, and survival rates in squamous cell carcinoma of the skin, ear, and lip: implications for treatment modality selection. *J Am Acad Dermatol.* 1992;26:976-990.

6. Garcia C, Holman J, Poletti E. Mohs surgery: commentaries and controversies. *Int J Dermatol.* 2005;44(11):893-905.

7. Bumsted RM, Ceilley RI, Panje WR, et al. Auricular malignant neoplasms. When is chemotherapy (Mohs' technique) necessary? *Arch Otolaryngol.* 1981;107:721-724.

8. Downes RN, Walker NPJ, Collin JRO. Micrographic (Mohs') surgery in the management of periocular basal cell epitheliomas. *Eye.* 1990;4:160-168.

9. Gill HS, Moscato EE, Seiff SR. Eyelid margin basal cell carcinoma managed with full-thickness en-face frozen section histopathology. *Ophthalmic Plast Reconstr Surg.* 2014;30(1):15-19.

10. Rossy KM, Lawrence N. Difficulty with surgical site identification: what role does it play in dermatology? *J Am Acad Dermatol.* 2012;67(2):257-261.

11. Lichtman MK, Countryman NB. Cell phone-assisted identification of surgery site. *Dermatol Surg.* 2013;39(3 Pt 1):491-492.

12. Neill BC, Billingsley EM. Light abrasion with a gauze pad for presurgical identification of skin cancer biopsy sites. *J Am Acad Dermatol.* 2021;85(4):e239-e240.

13. Ravitskiy L, Brodland DG, Zitelli JA. Cost analysis: Mohs micrographic surgery. *Dermatol Surg.* 2012;38(4):585-594.

14. Mansouri B, Bicknell LM, Hill D, Walker GD, Fiala K, Housewright C. Mohs micrographic surgery for the management of cutaneous malignancies. *Facial Plast Surg Clin North Am.* 2017;25(3):291-301.

15. Nassiripour L, Amirsadri M, Tabatabaeian M, Maracy MR. Cost-effectiveness of surgical excision versus Mohs micrographic surgery for nonmelanoma skin cancer: a retrospective cohort study. *J Res Med Sci.* 2016;21:91.

SECTION II
Surgical Considerations, Specimen Preparation, and Processing

4

Indications

Patrick Emanuel / Kevin G. Smith

Barriers
Indication Guidelines for MCS
The National Comprehensive Cancer Network
    Basal Cell Carcinoma
    Squamous Cell Carcinoma
    Melanoma
    Dermatofibrosarcoma Protuberans
    Merkel Cell Carcinoma
American Academy of Dermatology Appropriate
  Use Criteria

The Mohs Service Guidance and Standards
  (United Kingdom)
Cancer Staging Protocols
    American Joint Committee on Cancer
    Union for International Cancer Control
    Brigham and Women's Hospital
Summary

Margin control surgery (MCS) can be used in the management of practically any skin lesion, though in multifocal tumors or pathologies with a high incidence of satellite lesions, the importance of surgical margins is diminished. In these scenarios, MCS may serve as an adjunct to guide radical excision and reduce unnecessary morbidity.

BARRIERS

Before discussing indications, it is worth noting some key barriers to the utilization of MCS.

In his best-selling book *Thinking, Fast and Slow*, celebrated economist and psychologist Daniel Kahneman described two distinct ways, or paradigms, that our brains use to formulate decisions. In the first paradigm, we make decisions quickly, automatically, stereotypically, and unconsciously. This is the system that many surgeons typically use when excising a given skin tumor. They read the biopsy and histopathologic diagnosis and proceed briskly to a wide local excision (WLE) with the measured margin guideline detailed in a range of protocols. They've done this procedure many times before, they're familiar with its demands and confident that their experience will set them in good stead. In contrast, the second way that the brain formulates a decision is slow, effortful, logical, calculating, and conscious. This slow-thinking paradigm is more suitable when considering the many potentially complex aspects of MCS such as the available guidelines, the levels of the excision, coordination of the laboratory team, interpretation of the pathology and margin assessment, time constraints, as well as the integration of all these factors into a reconstruction plan. Human nature is always tempted to go with the fast system. It is knee-jerk, instinctual, and easier. Significant effort is required to resist this temptation and instead synthesize a surgical solution using the more measured contemplation of MCS.

Another barrier to MCS is the lack of facilities and appropriately trained specialists who can perform the procedure. Most pathology laboratories process frozen sections and routine skin excisions, but far fewer have the incentive or knowledge to process specimens with the level of precision needed for complete margin assessment. Similarly, surgeons tend to send a specimen off to the laboratory without a clear description of their expectations and may not understand the limits of traditional pathological margin assessment. To run an MCS service, a clear understanding of the entire process is ideal, and though perhaps daunting, this is achievable for most skin surgeons and pathology laboratories.

Constraints in funding and resources are unfortunately serious barriers in certain practice settings. Even in well-resourced settings, criteria have been defined as to when MCS is recommended or appropriate for common skin tumors. While a variety of different indication guidelines have been developed internationally, in many parts of the world there are no well-established criteria. In some countries, the national Mohs micrographic surgery (MMS) community has established criteria. Insurers and managers are eager to apply such guidelines when regulating access and making decisions to fund resource-intensive techniques.

For less common tumors, only limited guidelines for therapy exist. A rational approach is needed in these scenarios. In general, tumors that have a high recurrence rate, occur on cosmetically or functionally sensitive areas, and have a relatively cohesive growth should be considered for MCS.

INDICATION GUIDELINES FOR MCS

The commonly used documents detailing the indications for MCS are summarized here. The decision on which one to apply in a given practice is usually determined by geographic influences and personal preference.

THE NATIONAL COMPREHENSIVE CANCER NETWORK

The National Comprehensive Cancer Network (NCCN) is a not-for-profit alliance of 32 leading cancer centers in the United States devoted to patient care, research, and education. It periodically releases treatment guidelines by tumor type. The NCCN regards MMS and complete circumferential peripheral and deep margin assessment (CCPDMA)[a] as equivalent procedures provided that strict criteria are met to encourage equivalence in margin assessment (**Table 4.1**).

Basal Cell Carcinoma
The NCCN recommends MCS for "high-risk" basal cell carcinoma (BCCs)[1] (**Table 4.2**).

MCS is also recommended for low-risk BCCs which have positive histopathologic margins despite an excision with 4-mm clinical margins.

---

[a] CCPDMA is also called peripheral and deep *en face* margin assessment (PDEMA).

TABLE 4.1 Criteria for Definition of CCPDMA with NCCN
- The entire marginal surface of the specimen must be microscopically examined. This surface must include the radial and deep margin. - The specimen is orientated to allow mapping of positive margins. - Positive margins are re-excised, and the re-excised margin is also completely examined. - The time between steps must be rapid enough to prevent granulation of the wound as well as distortion, which confuses orientation.

TABLE 4.2 Features of High-Risk BCC	
Location	- Trunk, extremities >2 cm - Mask areas of the face, genitalia, hands, feet
Borders	Poorly defined
Immunosuppression	Present
Prior radiotherapy	Present
Perineural involvement	Present
Pathology	Infiltrative, micronodular, morpheaform, basosquamous, sclerosing, carcinosarcomatous

Squamous Cell Carcinoma

The NCCN recommends MCS for high-risk squamous cell carcinoma (SCCs) and very high-risk SCCs[2] (**Tables 4.3** and **4.4**).

Low-risk SCCs which have positive histopathologic margins despite an excision with 4-mm clinical margins are also recommended to have MCS.

The NCCN criteria are easy to apply in clinical practice and therefore are useful in defining risk.

One criticism of the NCCN has been the inclusion of a "poorly defined" border as a high-risk feature. A "poorly defined" border is a highly subjective metric that could be associated with many tumors, and as such it could be argued that in this case, the NCCN is currently too inclusive.

TABLE 4.3 Features of High-Risk SCC	
Location	- Trunk >2 cm to ≤4 cm - Head, neck, hands, feet, pretibial, anogenital
Borders	Poorly defined
Immunosuppression	Present
Prior radiotherapy	Present
Perineural involvement	Present
Recurrent	Yes
Rapid growth	Yes
Neurological symptoms	Yes
Histology	Acantholytic, adenosquamous, metaplastic subtypes

TABLE 4.4 Features of Very High-Risk SCC	
Size	>4 cm
Perineural involvement	Nerve invasion deeper than dermis or >0.1 mm
Depth of invasion	>6 mm or invasion beyond subcutis
Lymphatic or vascular involvement	Yes
Histology	Poorly differentiated, desmoplastic

Melanoma

MCS is not recommended in the NCCN criteria for invasive melanoma. It can be considered in melanoma in situ (MIS) and in minimally invasive melanoma where standard margins cannot be achieved given anatomic and functional constraints. When used, it should be performed along with a comprehensive histologic assessment of the tumor in paraffin. A key concept is that the margins are examined with MCS, but the central specimen (debulk) is submitted for routine paraffin sectioning.

Dermatofibrosarcoma Protuberans

MCS is the only surgical therapy for dermatofibrosarcoma protuberans (DFSP) recommended by the NCCN. Previously, WLE was suggested as a viable alternative, but this has since been removed. WLE is currently mentioned as an option if MCS is unavailable.[3]

Merkel Cell Carcinoma

MCS is considered appropriate by the NCCN. It is noted that a further safety margin dictated by the guidelines for wide local excision may be considered even when a complete margin assessment is performed. The key concept here is that there are no significant data on the use of MCS for Merkel cell carcinoma but its use makes sense conceptually.

AMERICAN ACADEMY OF DERMATOLOGY APPROPRIATE USE CRITERIA

In the United States, the American Academy of Dermatology released its comprehensive appropriate use criteria (see Chap. 3) for the use of MMS.

THE MOHS SERVICE GUIDANCE AND STANDARDS (UNITED KINGDOM)

In 2014, the British Association of Dermatologists formed a multidisciplinary group to determine the appropriateness of MMS in the United Kingdom.[4] This group formulated a set of standards. The main conclusion of the group was that MMS should only be used in cases of "complex" skin cancers. Different from the NCCN, complexity was defined as both a high-risk pathology and occurring within a high-risk anatomical site (**Table 4.5**).

For other cases with either high-risk pathology *or* high-risk site, MMS should be considered alongside alternative treatments such as radiotherapy.

CANCER STAGING PROTOCOLS

There is a variety of protocols to stratify the risk of skin cancers internationally. These can be useful in determining which cancers require special consideration for MCS. They are formulated by specialist groups and updated periodically to consider new research and data.

TABLE 4.5 UK Service Guidance and Standards for Mohs Micrographic Surgery Complexity Criteria

High-risk nonmelanoma skin cancers include:

- Recurrent and incompletely excised tumors following previous treatment including prior radiotherapy;
- When the cancer is large (often more than 2 cm);
- If the edges of the cancer are poorly defined (the clinician should aim to visualize with good illumination and magnification);
- Specific histological features associated with local recurrence, e.g., micronodular, morpheic/infiltrative, perineural, perivascular invasion;
- Cancers in immunosuppressed patients.

High-risk sites include those where preservation of healthy tissue is important for maintenance of function and physical appearance:

- Cancers in facial anatomical sites (H-Zone), e.g., eyelids, medial canthus, nasal tip and ala, preauricular area, ears, lips where preserving healthy tissue is critical to maintaining a person's skin function and physical appearance;
- Reconstruction involving the eyelid margins and immediate surrounding area is normally best undertaken by/with a recognized oculoplastic surgeon due to the sensitive nature of the periocular region and the risk of visual loss. Where this is not possible, surgery should be undertaken in close liaison with an ophthalmologist to safeguard ocular integrity;
- Thumb and fingers;
- Genitalia.

American Joint Committee on Cancer

The American Joint Committee on Cancer (AJCC) released its 8th edition in late 2016.[5] In contrast to previous versions, this edition specifically dealt with SCC of the head and neck skin. Risk of the primary tumor is in large part stratified by the clinical dimensions of the carcinoma (T1 $\leq$ 2 cm, T2 > 2 cm and $\leq$ 4 cm, T3 > 4 cm in greatest dimension). T1 and T2 tumors are upstaged if deep invasion and/or significant perineural invasion is present. Deep invasion is defined as tumors measuring more than 6 mm in thickness, or with invasion beyond subcutaneous fat. Significant perineural invasion is defined as invasion of subcutaneous nerves or larger dermal nerves (>0.1 mm in diameter).

BCC or adnexal tumors are not included within this staging protocol or in any part of the 8th edition of the AJCC. Nor is there a place for cutaneous SCC outside of the head and neck. It is tempting to also use the same metrics for non-head or neck cutaneous SCC for the sake of consistency, but it would be incorrect to apply the T staging to these tumors. Another criticism laid against this version of the AJCC is that a poorly differentiated or undifferentiated histopathology has not been included despite compelling evidence that this high-risk morphology is associated with poorer outcomes in low clinical stage AJCC tumours.[5]

Union for International Cancer Control

The Union for International Cancer Control (UICC) and AJCC work closely together and, in most instances, the tumor, node, metastasis (TNM) version of each organization is the same or very similar.[6] The key difference is that the UICC provides an additional chapter covering the trunk and limbs (titled "Carcinoma of the Skin"). This can also be applied to BCC and adnexal carcinoma rather than just SCC.

Brigham and Women's Hospital

The Brigham and Women's Hospital (BWH) staging system for skin cancer (**Table 4.6**) is quite similar to the 8th edition of the AJCC.[7] The main distinction is that poorly

TABLE 4.6 BWH Tumor Classification System

T1:	0 High-risk factors[†]
T2a:	1 High-risk factors
T2b:	2-3 High-risk factors
T3:	4 High-risk factors *or* bone invasion

[†]*High-risk factors include clinical diameter ≥2 cm, poorly differentiated histology, perineural invasion ≥0.1 mm, invasion beyond subcutaneous fat.*

differentiated histopathology is included as a risk factor. Many physicians prefer to apply this system because it seems to stratify risk well, is not regularly changed, and relies on remembering the logical risk factors.

SUMMARY

There is a range of available guidelines to help the physician decide which patients would be appropriate for MCS. Staging protocols are used to determine risk and therefore can be applied to the triage of those tumors for which MCS may be considered optimal therapy. It's all well and good having these as a filter to the procedure but it requires intent and effort on the part of the clinical team to implement the systems to perform the procedure. And, of course, the resources need to be available.

References

1. National Comprehensive Cancer Network. Basal Cell Skin Cancer (Version 1.2021). https://www.nccn.org/professionals/physician_gls/pdf/nmsc.pdf. Accessed August 12, 2021.
2. National Comprehensive Cancer Network. Squamous Cell Skin Cancer (Version 1.2021). https://www.nccn.org/professionals/physician_gls/pdf/squamous.pdf. Accessed August 12, 2021.
3. National Comprehensive Cancer Network. Dermatofibrosarcoma Protuberans (Version 2.2022). https://www.nccn.org/guidelines/guidelinesdetail?category=1&id=1430. Accessed May 25, 2022.
4. British Association of Dermatology. Service Standards. https://www.bad.org.uk/health-care-professionals/clinical-services/service-guidance/mohs. Accessed August 12, 2021.
5. Thompson AK, Kelley BF, Prokop LJ, Murad MH, Baum CL. Risk factors for cutaneous squamous cell carcinoma recurrence, metastasis, and disease-specific death: a systematic review and meta-analysis. *JAMA Dermatol.* 2016;152(4):419-428.
6. Sobin L, Gospodarowicz M, Wittekind C, eds. *UICC International Union Against Cancer TNM Classification of Malignant Tumors.* 7th ed. West Sussex, United Kingdom: Wiley-Blackwell; 2009.
7. Karia PS, Jambusaria-Pahlajani A, Harrington DP, Murphy GF, Qureshi AA, Schmults CD. Evaluation of American Joint Committee on Cancer, International Union Against Cancer, and Brigham and Women's Hospital tumor staging for cutaneous squamous cell carcinoma. *J Clin Oncol.* 2014;32(4):327-334.

5

Surgical Technique and Specimen Mapping

Mark Izzard / Patrick Emanuel

To the Death of Guesswork
The Biopsy
Debulk
Clinical Marking
Levels and Mapping
    What Is a Level?
    Mapping
The First Level
    Intent
        Attempting to Remove the Tumor with
            the First Level
        Not Attempting to Remove the Tumor
            with the First Level
    Standard Ring First Level

How Deep to Go?
Orientation Notches and Inking
The Bevel
Second and Subsequent Levels
    Further Resection Strategies
        Complete Ring (Nontargeted Resection)
        Portion of the Margin (Targeted Resection)
Concepts of MCS for Tumors with a Highly
Infiltrative Pattern or Multifocal Growth
    Evaluating Tumor Size
    Behavior at the Margin
    Safety Margins
    Tissue-Sparing
Summary

TO THE DEATH OF GUESSWORK

Surgical oncology is to some extent a form of brinkmanship. The surgeon is juggling morbidity versus clearance every time a cancer is resected. While every tumor is "resectable," it is often a matter of morbidity and mortality. For surgical outcomes, surgeons tend to focus on avoiding positive margins rather than over-resecting tumors and creating large defects. This is for good reason given that a missed positive margin can be devastating if not fatal for patients. However, making large holes for small tumors can likewise have devastating effects, particularly for lesions on the face where ongoing morbidity from neurovascular fallout, loss of function, and altered cosmesis can have a huge impact on patients' lives. A technique where only the tumor is removed with a narrow—but clear—margin causing minimal morbidity has remained the holy grail for surgical oncologists. Margin control surgery (MCS) is the closest we have to achieving this in treating skin cancer.

Surgical brinkmanship comes in the form of educated *guesswork*. Tumors can be resected via two distinct philosophies:

- *To operate to anatomy.* The surgeon removes an entire unit that encompasses the tumor.
- *To operate to pathology.* The surgeon estimates the clinical margin of a tumor and the excision aims to excise just this.

Operating to anatomy is quite nuanced. In surgical oncology, lung cancers are a good example. With a pneumonectomy, instead of leaving behind a nonfunctioning lung and risking positive margins, it is often wiser to remove the whole lung lobe. Similarly, when dealing with a large basal cell carcinoma (BCC) on the nasal alar—occupying more than 50% of the alar—the surgeon will remove the entire alar skin to reconstruct the defect as per the subunit approach, so why not just remove the subunit as the first level? This approach is not tissue-sparing but usually removes the entire lesion with the first attempt.

These philosophies involve some form of *guesswork*. The central tenant of MCS is not to spare tissue or remove lesions in their entirety, it is to *avoid guesswork*.

THE BIOPSY

All lesions undergoing MCS need a biopsy to confirm the diagnosis prior to a surgical procedure. This is usually done at the preassessment appointment; however, depending on necessity, biopsies of non-melanocytic lesions can be performed on the day of the surgery with a frozen section. Biopsy adds little morbidity or cost to the patient.

While an excisional biopsy is always a pathologist's preference, this is not feasible for many lesions. Choosing whether to do a shave, curettage, punch, or surgical incisional biopsy is key and depends on the pathology, anatomic site, and patient factors (e.g., coagulation or healing issues). Without a reasonable understanding of skin pathology, the surgeon is not equipped to choose the appropriate method.

Generally, curettage should be reserved for BCCs or low-risk squamous cell carcinoma (SCCs) where the microscopic thickness and other staging parameters are less relevant. In addition to diagnosis, curettage has the added benefits of approximating the tumor's size before excision and facilitating manipulation of the excision specimen in the laboratory (**Fig. 5.1**).

Generally, shave biopsies are good for superficial lesions in which viewing maximum epidermis is ideal for the diagnosis (e.g., thin melanocytic lesions, superficial BCCs, SCCs in situ: see **Figs. 5.2** and **5.3**). Shave biopsies are particularly helpful for flat atypical, pigmented lesions on cosmetically sensitive skin as they provide far more epidermis and therefore diagnostic information for the pathologist when compared with punch biopsies. The distinction between solar lentigo, pigmented actinic keratosis, and melanoma is almost always possible with this type of biopsy. It can be argued that shave biopsies risk transecting the thickness of a tumor and impeding the ability to measure its thickness, but this almost never occurs when dealing with flat lesions where there is no suspicion of deep dermal invasion. It is important to also remember that thin invasive melanomas are very thin anatomically (less than 0.8-mm thick), which is often well within the limits of the depth of a shave biopsy.

Punch biopsies are often used for thicker BCCs and SCCs. Punch biopsies of melanocytic lesions should be discouraged as it is often impossible to get a good idea of the lesion's architecture and misdiagnosis can occur. Deeper incisional surgical biopsies are appropriate for some thicker BCCs, SCCs, and suspected invasive melanomas in which an excisional biopsy is not feasible.

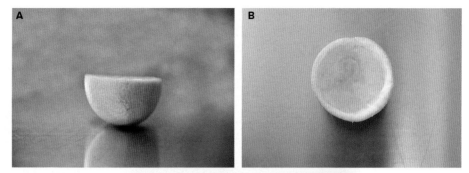

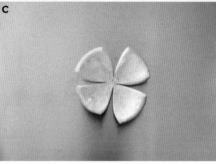

FIGURE 5.1. **A-C: Curettage essentially scoops out the tumor leaving the "rind" or margin behind in the patient, rather like hollowing out an orange (A, B).** Curettage can give a rough estimate of the tumor size and shape which is helpful when choosing the size of the surgical excision. The rind left behind is easier to manipulate and flatten, allowing examination of the entire margin in one plane (C).

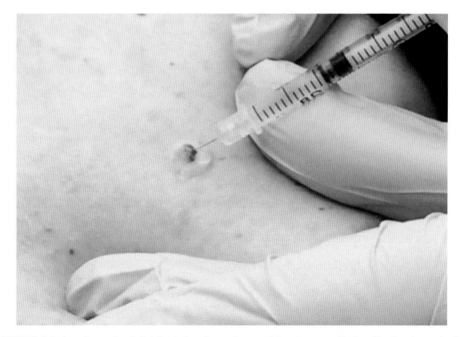

FIGURE 5.2. **Local anesthesia is injected under and around the pigmented lesion.** The local anesthetic raises the lesion which facilitates the shave biopsy.

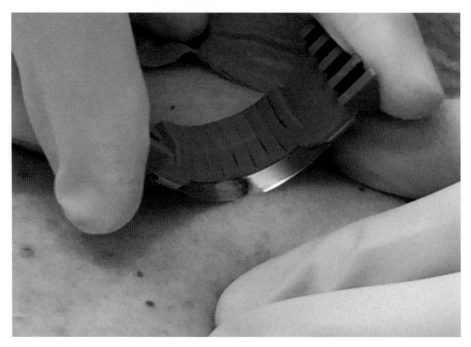

FIGURE 5.3. **A wide variety of scalpels can be used for the shave biopsies.** Small lesions like this can aim for full removal of the clinical extent of the pigmented lesion. Larger lesions can be partially sampled. The idea is to get maximum epidermis in the biopsy, allowing the pathologist to assess the architecture of the lesion and maximizing the chance of a correct diagnosis. With this technique, no suture needs to be removed and if the diagnosis turns out to be benign, the cosmetic outcome is often superior to that of a punch biopsy.

It is worth re-emphasizing that there is significant nuance in factoring in anatomic and patient factors when choosing the biopsy type.

DEBULK

A debulk specimen aims to remove the bulk of the tumor before the margin assessment steps. Debulk can take the form of a curettage or a scalpel debulk. Scalpel debulk is useful for tumors in which staging is important (e.g., melanoma) and cases in which the biopsy may not be representative of the whole tumor. Curettage debulk is useful for low-risk tumors where it helps define the extent of the tumor and facilitates specimen processing. The debulk specimen is usually sent to the pathology laboratory in formalin for regular paraffin processing.

CLINICAL MARKING

Clinical marking is an attempt to estimate the size and shape of the lesion. Usually, a 1-mm rim is drawn around the identified tumor, but this depends on the tumor type and the intent of the surgeon. A dermatoscope is very useful for this process. Difficulties arise in lesions with significant background actinic dysplasia or inflammatory changes (e.g., due to rosacea).

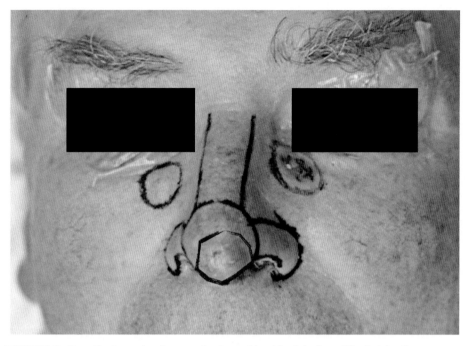

FIGURE 5.4. **Once the tumor has been excised, considerable distortion of the facial units may occur due to relaxing of the underlying connective tissues.** Preoperative marking is always useful in assessing and planning reconstruction.

Because the whole margin will be examined, where there is uncertainty it is helpful to undersize the excision and the positive margins will serve to guide the subsequent excisions. Contrary to the practice of many surgeons, in MCS it is acceptable to cut through a tumor. The idea of curetting out or cutting through tumor while still in situ in the patient can be quite challenging for those accustomed to *en bloc* tumor resections but there is no evidence that this process leads to tumor seeding or embolic events.

It is helpful to draw on the local subsites that are adjacent to the tumor. If the tumor transgresses subsites, the next is drawn and so on (**Fig. 5.4**).

LEVELS AND MAPPING

What Is a Level?

Level is the term used to describe surgical removal of tissue during MCS that is prepared and examined in order to look at the whole margin of the resected tissue. It is not a biopsy, nor a debulk, nor a safety margin. *Layer* is the preferred term in some communities.

It helps to think of a level in geological terms. Imagine we are digging a hole, with each level of earth revealing new information about the terrain around us as we go down level by level (**Fig. 5.5**). Hence the term.

Mapping

Now imagine that we are on an archeological dig and looking for an artifact buried within that soil (**Fig. 5.6**). With each descending level, we start to map the area and get an idea of the dimensions, depth, and size of the site we are excavating. As the procedure advances,

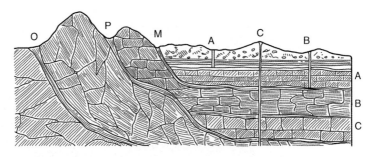

FIGURE 5.5. The level can involve digging deeper or digging outwards or both as the site is explored.

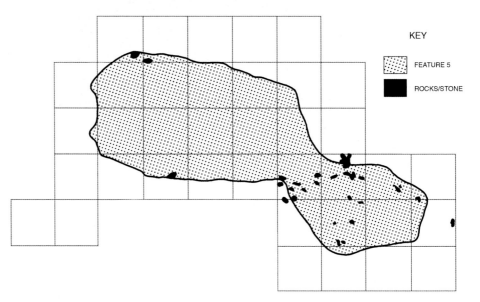

FIGURE 5.6. **An archeological dig site is like an MCS map.** Notice that the squares around the perimeter contain no additional features, just as the periphery of a completely excised tumor will have no tumor at the margin. Also, like archeology, a key trick in MCS is knowing where to start digging.

each mapped area gives us an indication of where to dig next. By the time it is finished, we have a full map of the entire area and the whole site has been excavated, and nothing relevant remains in the surrounding soil. This principle of mapping also applies in MCS.

Any time a level of tissue is removed in MCS, the tumor is mapped onto a mapping sheet. Mapping is a physical process that involves a pencil and paper. This may seem old-fashioned in our era of paperless everything, but none of the electronic processes have so far proved themselves superior in terms of accuracy and efficiency. Mapping in both MCS and archeology requires meticulous attention and additional time when compared to doing a blind archeological site dig or a regular wide local excision (WLE).

THE FIRST LEVEL

The *first level* is the first excision of the tumor. The first level is excised, orientated, and processed for complete histopathologic assessment of the margin and mapping. The size of the first level depends to a degree on the *intent* of the surgeon.

Intent

As with many things in life, we must know what we want to achieve before we can act.

The ethos behind taking the first level is twofold and distinct:

ATTEMPTING TO REMOVE THE TUMOR WITH THE FIRST LEVEL. At first glance, this may seem obvious, as opposed to not trying to remove the tumor on the first attempt, but they are two very different concepts that lead to two very different surgical techniques. Who would not want to remove the tumor with the first level? Well, attempting to remove the tumor on the first attempt is an expression of intent.

Attempting to remove the tumor with the first level could mean: I'm trying to remove the tumor with the first level and I don't care about how much normal tissue I take.

Or: I'm trying to remove the tumor with the first level and I'm trying not to take too much normal tissue.

The purpose of the first level could be to use a WLE margin or an anatomical margin and then examine the entire margin histologically to ensure it is clear. *This is non-tissue-sparing.* The purpose of the MCS here is to ensure clear margins before primary reconstruction. The surgeon is saying, "I'm taking a standard WLE margin as proposed in the medical literature, hoping to do just the one level, but I'm going to check it's clear before I do a complex flap or graft reconstruction."

Consider these two scenarios in dealing with a standard BCC:

- A 5-mm clinical margin will clear the tumor approximately 95% of the time. If the surgeon employed MCS at the time of removal, they would avoid needing to re-excise a reconstruction for 5% of their resections. Here the surgeon is intending to get the lesion out on the first attempt. *There is no consideration given to tissue-sparing.* The margin assessment is purely to add confidence that the reconstruction can primarily go ahead. This is quite different from the way most margin control surgeons routinely practice. The key advantage of this technique is a much lower number of positive first levels, thereby saving money and time. Disadvantages would be a larger defect and a larger reconstruction with more patient morbidity.
- Another option is to use a narrow excision margin and then use the MCS to see if the entire margin is clear. *This is tissue-sparing.* Here the surgeon is trying to remove the lesion with the smallest margin possible. Where this is useful is in well-defined tumors such as nodular BCCs and well-differentiated SCCs. In experienced hands, a clear margin can be obtained with first level approximately 75% of the time with a 1-mm margin or less of normal tissue. The advantages of this technique are a smaller defect and a smaller reconstruction with less patient morbidity. Disadvantages are a higher number of positive first levels and a higher cost in terms of money and time.

NOT ATTEMPTING TO REMOVE THE TUMOR WITH THE FIRST LEVEL. Sometimes the aim of the first level is not to attempt to remove the tumor entirely.

Rather like the archeology map, the edges of the lesion are explored by mapping the tumor with levels. With diffuse or hard-to-see tumors such as amelanotic melanoma in situ or some dermatofibrosarcoma protuberans (DFSPs), the true edges of the lesion are invisible to the naked eye. The first level may start in the middle of the lesion with a rough estimation of clinically apparent edge, although the surgeon makes no attempt to clear the lesion. Radial contiguous excisions are performed until the margins start to become apparent. This is usually performed by the ring technique explained later in this chapter. This is true MCS, often requiring multiple levels, and it may be time-consuming and expensive.

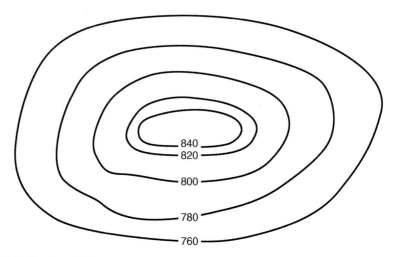

FIGURE 5.7. **The shape of the tissue ring mirrors the tumor, like a contour map.**

Standard Ring First Level

In a standard ring first level, a margin is drawn around the visible tumor. Here, "ring" does not mean circular but a circumferential and deep complete margin. The size of the margin from visible tumor depends on the intent of the clearance (**Fig. 5.7**). If the tumor is round, the ring is round, and a lozenge-shaped tumor calls for a lozenge-shaped ring. The idea is to leave out as much normal tissue as possible as it keeps the level smaller, easier, and faster for processing.

How Deep to Go?

This is a common issue that often comes up with trainees. Again, it combines assessment of the tumor clinically with information from the biopsy (**Fig. 5.8**). If the bulk of the tumor has been removed with a debulking curettage, it is often easier to judge the depth of excision needed. In some scenarios, the true depth of invasion only becomes clear when the first level is examined microscopically.

Orientation Notches and Inking

One of the fundamentals of mapping is orientation. Just as a regular map is useless without an indication of the north, so too is an MCS map without a "patient locator." This is key to keeping things simple and standardized. Most errors in MCS come about from loss of orientation, from the notch placement, inking, or reversing the specimen. Of importance when orientating the specimen and preventing marking and interpretation errors is to orientate the specimen to the patient.

Any number of notches can be used. Often it is two notches, 90° apart, with one "primary" notch orientated to the vertex of the patient or the "top" and the other at 90° to it (**Fig. 5.9**). The top can be called the 12 o'clock notch. The 12 o'clock notch at the top or vertex is blue (think: "the blue sky above"). The other notch is red or orange or green depending on preference. The notches are placed after a circumferential incision is made in the skin. They cross both the specimen and the residual skin (**Fig. 5.10**).

Once the specimen is removed, it is handed off to nursing or laboratory staff on a moist swab with an orientation dot drawn on it. Aligning the 12 o'clock notch to the orientation dot makes inking easier and minimizes error (**Fig. 5.11**). Though the specimen can often

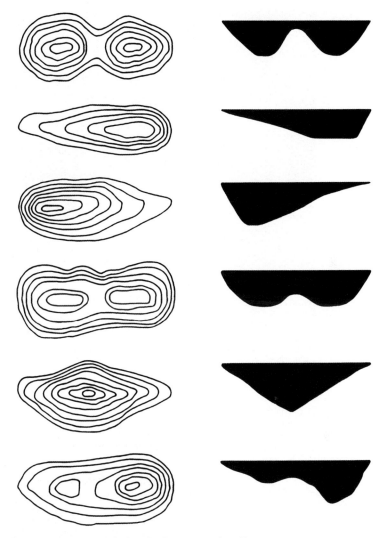

FIGURE 5.8. There are many variations in the topography of how tumors grow.

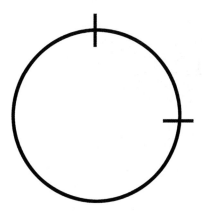

FIGURE 5.9. The reason for the two notches 90° apart is that it makes it impossible to confuse the orientation. The second notch will be at either 3 o'clock or 9 o'clock depending on the anatomy. The notch crosses onto the patient's skin to help the surgeon locate where a further excision is needed when the level is positive.

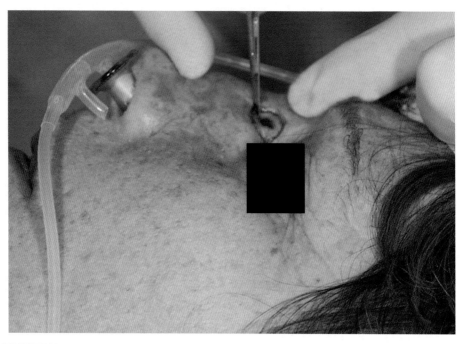

FIGURE 5.10. **Notches are placed after a circumferential incision is made in the skin.** They cross both the specimen and the residual skin so positive areas can be easily located on the patient.

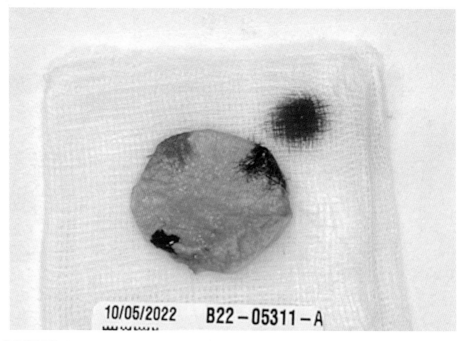

FIGURE 5.11. **A moist swab with an orientation dot (black in this case) is used to transport the specimen to the lab.** It can be helpful to point the 12 o'clock notch to the dot on the gauze for ease of inking. In this case, three colors were used for orientation.

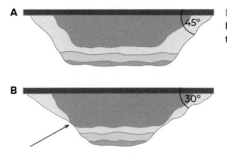

FIGURE 5.12. (A, B): These diagrams show how a flat bevel angle can risk undercutting and exposing the tumor.

be processed in one tissue block, some surgeons prefer cutting the specimen into quadrants and processing these as separate specimens to aid in orientation.

The Bevel

As is outlined further in Chap. 6 (Specimen Preparation), the bevel is important in processing the level in the laboratory. A bevel of 45° or steeper to vertical is usually ideal when the specimen is to be processed using the Mohs method. When other methods are used in the laboratory, a regular 90° excision is usually appropriate. Communication with the technician preparing the slides is key. It is important to not make the bevel too shallow, as this risks undercutting the tumor (**Fig. 5.12**).

The defect following the first level is dressed with a hemostatic substance and a pressure dressing is applied. Further oral or local anesthetic may be administered while the patient waits for the slide processing.

SECOND AND SUBSEQUENT LEVELS

The map of the first level is used to indicate if and where there is a positive margin. If any part of the level is positive, more tissue needs to be excised to clear the tumor. This is called the *second level*. If the second level is also positive, a *third level* is taken, and so on until clearance is achieved. Notching and inking of these specimens is carried out in the same fashion as for the first level.

Further Resection Strategies

The levels after the first level can take many forms. These can be split into *nontargeted* and *targeted* resections. For nontargeted resections, the only pertinent information is that the margin is positive, so a wider nontargeted excision is performed without paying attention to orientation.

COMPLETE RING (NONTARGETED RESECTION). In an effort to keep things simple and avoid mistakes, one way to proceed following a positive first level is to remove a further complete ring of tissue. This is particularly popular with surgeons just starting out in their MCS practice, particularly if the lesion is small. If the deep margin is clear in the first level, this nontargeted second level will just be circumferential and not include the deep margin (**Fig. 5.13**). If the tumor is positive diffusely radially and at the deep margin in the first level, then a further complete ring of tissue, deep and radial margin is needed.

This technique usually does not end up being very tissue-sparing. It does, however, eliminate *guesswork*, and prevents errors of orientation, overlap, and gaps.

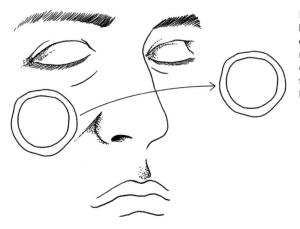

FIGURE 5.13. A nontargeted second level may include a complete ring excision of the margin. The entire ring is embedded *en face* and examined histologically. This is not as tissue-sparing as a targeted second level but is less prone to error.

PORTION OF THE MARGIN (TARGETED RESECTION). More commonly, the map of the first level is used to guide a subsequent *targeted* resection. Here the surgeon uses the map to tailor the subsequent resection to the specific tumor that is mapped (**Fig. 5.14**). This technique relies on very accurate mapping and orientation notches at reference points on the patient.

For these targeted resections, there are a few possibilities as to what needs to be achieved based on the positive margins seen in the first level:

- A further complete ring of tissue, radial margin only (the tumor was positive diffusely radially in the first level)
- A portion or portions of margins, some of the radial margin, and/or some of the deep margin (the tumor was positive in some areas radially and deep in the first level)
- Deep margin only, no radial margin (the tumor was present at the deep margin in the first level)

The concern here is of course that some tumors may be left behind so careful attention is needed when correlating the mapped positive margin with the defect on the patient.

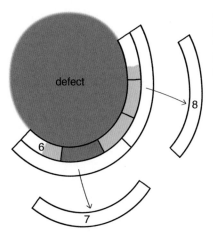

FIGURE 5.14. In this example, a portion of the first level is positive radially (approximately 1-8 o'clock). The second (targeted) level is also positive (approximately 2-7 o'clock). The third level (tissue blocks marked 7 and 8) is negative.

CONCEPTS OF MCS FOR TUMORS WITH A HIGHLY INFILTRATIVE PATTERN OR MULTIFOCAL GROWTH

One of the criticisms leveled at MCS is the inability to deal with tumors that have a highly infiltrative pattern *or* a noncontiguous growth pattern with foci of tumor breaking away from the main body of the tumor.

When an infiltrative front is seen microscopically, there are a few possibilities as to what it may mean:

- It could be an artifact of processing and not authentic microsatellite growth. A very infiltrative tumor may be cross-cut so that an island or nests appear to be isolated from the main body of the tumor when they are not. This is commonly seen in DFSP. It may also be seen in melanoma, Merkel cell carcinoma, and highly infiltrative SCC or BCC.
- Tumor microsatellites are occurring. Classic cutaneous tumors associated with this phenomenon include Merkel cell carcinoma, angiosarcoma, in situ sebaceous carcinoma, and melanoma. Conceptually, however, any malignancy capable of metastasizing has the potential to grow in this fashion, and high-risk SCC and BCC may rarely show this feature.
- The tumor is truly multifocal (either inherently or due to tumor recurrence).

If the tumor truly is discontiguous, an excision margin can be negative for malignancy but there may be deposits of malignancy outside of the margin. A false clearance will lead to a recurrence. This is a potential issue for any discontiguous tumor, regardless of the size of the margin excised, but the confidence of clearance increases as the margin size increases. Discussion of these cases at a multidisciplinary meeting (MDM) for the possible use of adjunct therapies (e.g., radiotherapy) should be considered.

For all of these malignancies, whether prone to microsatellites or highly infiltrative, the literature recommends taking wide margins guided by the assessment of the clinical margin. However, this is a crude metric for these tumors and ignores patient morbidity.

The concepts of MCS in this scenario include:

1. Evaluating tumor size
2. Evaluating the pattern/behavior at the margin
3. Taking a safety margin
4. Tissue-sparing

Evaluating Tumor Size

Instead of excising highly infiltrative tumors with the large margins upfront (e.g., 3-5 cm), a narrow margin is drawn (e.g., 2 mm) around the clinical visible tumor and the margin is excised and examined to assess what is happening. If the entire circumference is positive, then it is much more likely that the tumor is large. However, as is often the case, the tumor may be positive in just one region and we thus have some initial idea of tumor size (**Figs. 5.15** and **5.16**).

Behavior at the Margin

A positive margin at MCS can give us information about the pattern of infiltration and extent of positivity (**Fig. 5.17**). Once we get a positive margin, further excisions can aim to either target just the positive area *or* continue with another complete ring. With highly infiltrative or possibly discontiguous tumors, it is usually wise to continue with the ring approach. If so, the ring approach is continued until the whole margin is negative for malignancy (**Fig. 5.18**).

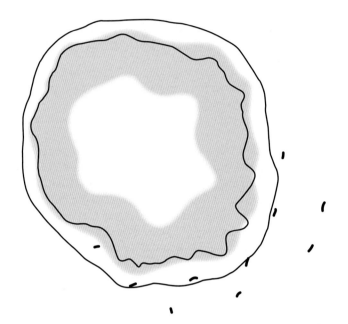

FIGURE 5.15. The first level reveals that the tumor (black dots) is extending radially in one area.

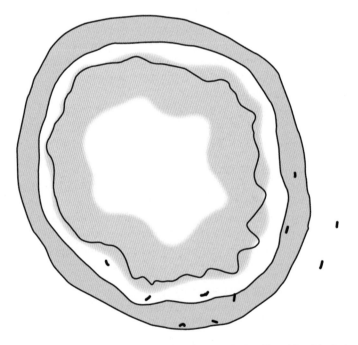

FIGURE 5.16. A second ring is taken and shows that the margin is still positive (black dots) in this area.

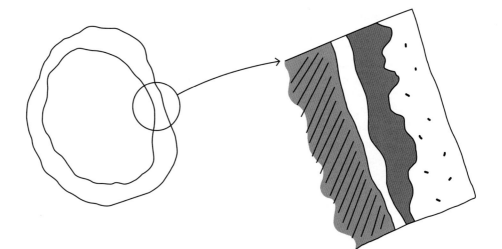

FIGURE 5.17. Histologic examination of the margin reveals the pattern of invasion. Multiple areas or microscopic tumors with infiltration of native structures (e.g., nerves) should alert the surgeon to take wider margins.

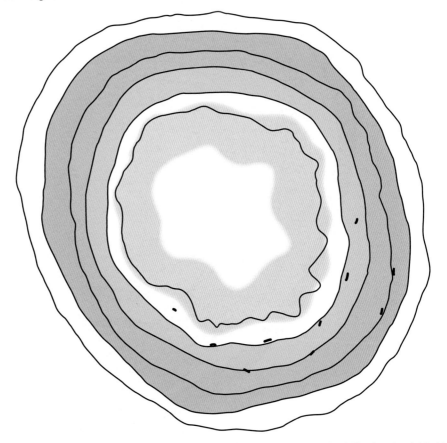

FIGURE 5.18. Dots of tumor remain at the margin as further rings are excised. The last ring (white) is negative for malignancy.

Safety Margins

When the ring is entirely negative for malignancy, proceeding with a safety margin is often the next step.

What is a safety margin? A safety margin is a rim of normal tissue removed around the wound following MCS. This margin is processed in paraffin and processed so the whole margin is examined (**Fig. 5.19**). Theoretically, these should always be negative for malignancy, but they have a specific utility when treating difficult and unusual cases. Safety margins are often taken during MCS for discontiguous tumors, highly infiltrative tumors, and tumors with a subtle histopathology that can be difficult to see with frozen section slides.

As the safety margin offers the chance to examine the specimen in paraffin sections, the slides are much easier for the pathologist to interpret. In addition, the wide range of immunohistochemical studies available to the pathologist can be used on this safety margin to assure complete excision.

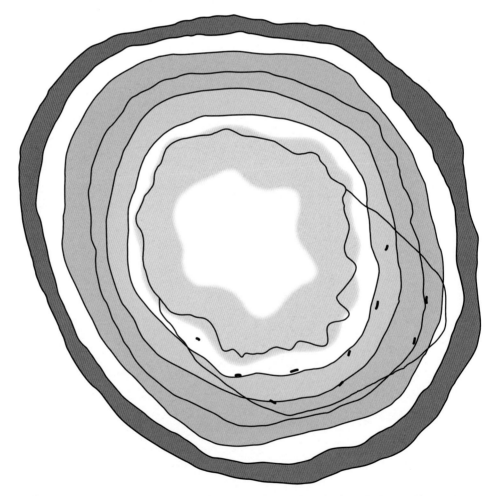

FIGURE 5.19. The safety margin (shown in red) is excised and sent in formalin for paraffin histology. Only after complete excision are we able to see the shape of the tumor (border roughly drawn in black).

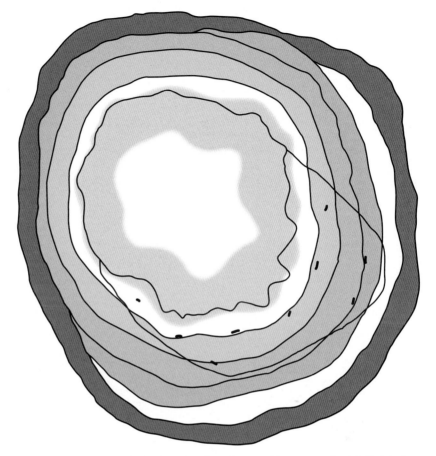

FIGURE 5.20. The safety margin is taken, but tissue is spared from approximately 7 o'clock around to 1 o'clock.

Tissue-Sparing

Rather than complete rings, another option is to map the tumor more precisely and spare tissue (**Fig. 5.20**).

Reasons for this tissue-sparing approach are varied and include:

- The number of levels already taken (as described above) gives good confidence of clearance.
- An organ or anatomic reason in which the risks of tissue-sparing do not outweigh the benefits.
- A delayed closure will be performed, so waiting for the final safety margin pathology result is feasible.

SUMMARY

The intent of the surgeon plays an integral role in formulating a surgical strategy that avoids *guesswork*. The chosen biopsy, debulk, and excision methods depend largely on the nature of the pathology and involve balancing the successful excision and practical considerations with patient morbidity.

6

Specimen Preparation

Patrick Emanuel / Mark Izzard

Specimen Orientation
Inking
Six Main Specimen Processing Techniques
   The Bread Loaf Technique (Serial
     Transverse Vertical Cross-Sections)
   Mohs Technique (*En Face* Horizontal
     Sectioning)
   En Face 3D Technique

The Munich Technique
Perimeter Technique
Peripheral Sectioning of Wedge Excisions
Debulk Considerations
Safety Margins
Specific Processing Issues
Summary

What happens to a skin excision specimen after it disappears out of the operating room is a mystery to many surgeons. But some surgeons realize that a basic understanding of pathology is often needed to make informed surgical decisions. And some surgeons (usually dermatologists) are so interested in the pathology processing that they take on the role of the pathologist themselves.

SPECIMEN ORIENTATION

There is tremendous variation in how specimens are orientated when they reach the laboratory. Communication between the pathologist and surgeon is key in arriving at a satisfactory protocol to allow uniformity in processing. Larger specimens are often orientated with the placement of sutures, but a simpler option is the cutting of small notches by the surgeon (as outlined in Chap. 5). A single orientation at the top of the specimen is generally sufficient because once you know where superior is, then inferior, medial, and lateral can be deduced. Where precise mapping is more critical, more than one notch or suture may be used for orientation.

INKING

The specimen is inked using Indian ink and this information is drawn on a corresponding map. Inking can be done by the surgeon in the procedure room or by the pathologist or histotechnician (**Fig. 6.1**). Some surgeons prefer to do the inking in the procedure room to reduce the chance of placing ink on the wrong margins.

The processing technique chosen will determine the inking method. Anywhere from one to eight colors may be used. Whichever method is chosen, it needs to be understood that the

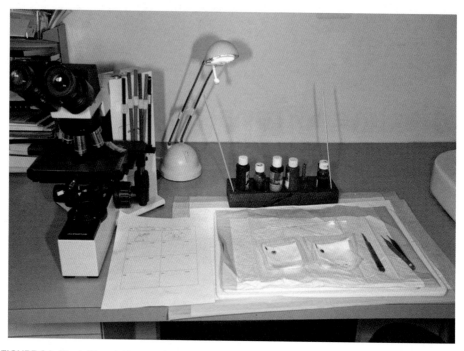

FIGURE 6.1. The inking station needs to be well-lit and clean. The specimen map is drawn with the corresponding notches and colors.

expectation of the inking process is that it will permit the localization of any positive margin microscopically so that positive margins can be located and re-excised on the patient.

Care needs to be taken not to use too much ink as the ink may inadvertently bleed and confuse the margins. The same problem can also occur if the specimen is too wet. The quality of the ink is also important, as poor-quality ink may wash off during the tissue preparation.

SIX MAIN SPECIMEN PROCESSING TECHNIQUES

Though there are further permutations, the main aspects of processing skin specimens for margin control surgery (MCS) can be boiled down to six distinct methods. Deciding which one to use depends on the size of the excision, the pathology, and the preference of the staff involved. It is important to mention that all these methods can be performed with intraoperative frozen sections or formalin-fixed paraffin sections (slow Mohs).

The Bread Loaf Technique (Serial Transverse Vertical Cross-Sections)

This technique does not allow for the examination of the entire margin, regardless of how meticulously it is managed (**Figs. 6.2** to **6.6**). The specimen is inked along the entirety of the surgical margin rather than just as an orientating dot at the specimen pole. It is cut vertically (perpendicular to the epidermis rather than horizontally) along its short axis and the pieces of tissue are embedded vertically so that vertical sections are produced for microscopic examination.

It is difficult to determine what percentage of the margin is evaluated with this technique. Various percentages are quoted, with the most scathing reviews of the bread loaf

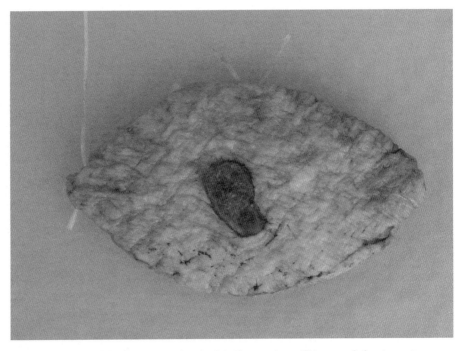

FIGURE 6.2. **The excision has sutures to orientate the specimen.** This example has two sutures. Though sutures are commonly used, orientating notches cut by the surgeon are generally easier to manage. Often, only one orientating suture or notch is needed. For example, with a single suture indicating superior, the other margins can be extrapolated. More precise orientation may need more notches.

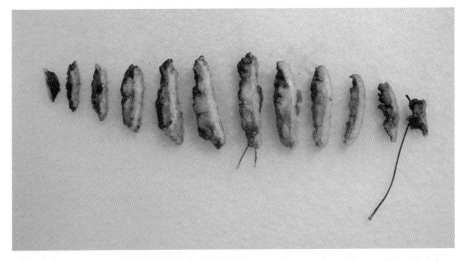

FIGURE 6.3. **For the bread loaf technique, two colors are usually used, and these will meet at the "spine" of the excision's deep margin.** The specimen is cut vertically in 2-mm-thick sections. Other protocols remove the tips of the ellipse, but for the purposes of margin assessment, the entire specimen is cut in the same way.

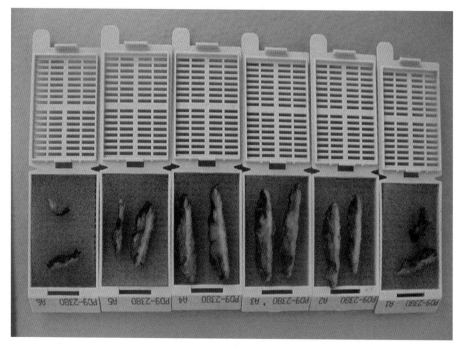

FIGURE 6.4. The tissue is placed into cassettes ready for embedding.

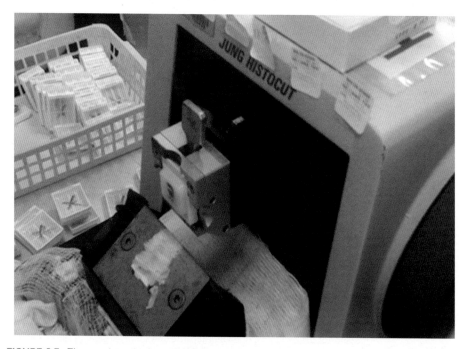

FIGURE 6.5. The specimen in the paraffin block is cut with a microtome to produce slides which are then stained with hematoxylin and eosin.

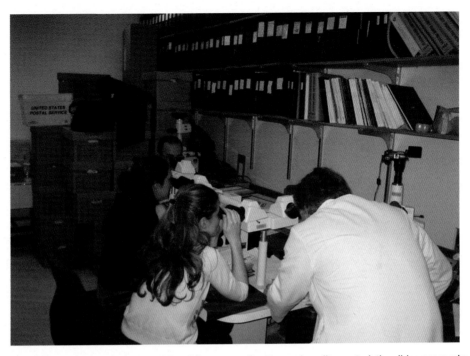

FIGURE 6.6. Following staining of the slides, cover-slipping, and quality control, the slides are ready for examination with the microscope.

technique claiming that the method examines less than 1% of the entire surgical margin.[1,2] There are several variables to consider in arriving at this estimation, such as the thickness of the bread-loafed sections in the cassette, the amount of tissue discarded between each level that gets mounted onto a slide, the thickness of each section, and the number of sections obtained.

Partial margin sampling would not be a major issue if all skin tumors grew in a predictable, symmetrical way. Systematic geometric analyses have shown us that skin tumors frequently have irregular infiltrative borders and grow with small extensions or "tentacles" which are missed when the specimen is cut with the bread loaf method (**Fig. 6.7**). This is borne out in clinical practice: In a study looking at excisions of facial basal cell carcinoma (BCCs) excised with 2-mm margins, it was found that bread-loafing the specimen is only 44% sensitive for identifying residual tumor at the surgical margin.[3-5] For smaller excisions, the accuracy is even lower. In a study looking at BCC shave excisions which were reported to have negative margins, an immediate wider excision was thoroughly examined and showed the residual tumor in 78.4% of cases.[6]

Some pathologists favor the bread loaf technique as it allows accurate measurement of the thickness of tumor (**Fig. 6.8**) and enables an assessment of the relationship of the tumor to the margin. When tissue is embedded horizontally or if the margins are removed and examined separately, margin measurements are impossible and the surgeon does not know if the tumor is millimeters or centimeters from the margin. The bread loaf technique is also technically easier to perform. Key features of the bread loaf technique are highlighted in **Table 6.1**.

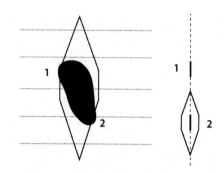

FIGURE 6.7. **The bread loaf method only examines a portion of the margin.** Here, the tumor involves the radial margin in areas 1 and 2. These areas are not represented in the sections examined microscopically and consequently there is persistent tumor along the closed wound site. The black area is the tumor. The solid line is the surgical excision. The dotted lines are the cross-sections used for bread-loafing. The dashed line is the surgical scar. (Reproduced with permission from Kimyai-Asadi A, Goldberg LH, Jih MH. Accuracy of serial transverse cross-sections in detecting residual basal cell carcinoma at the surgical margins of an elliptical excision specimen. *J Am Acad Dermatol.* 2005;53(3):469-474.[3])

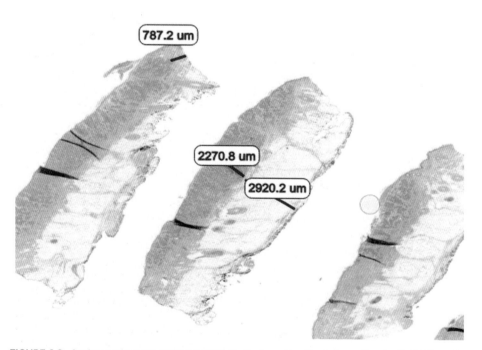

FIGURE 6.8. **As the sections are cut vertically with the bread loaf technique, the depth (thickness) of the tumor can be measured, as can the deep and radial margins.** However, as the deep and radial margins represented in the sections comprise only a fraction of the entire margin, these margin measurements are likely inaccurate.

TABLE 6.1 Key Features of Bread Loaf Method		
Examines entire margin	Can measure distance to margin	Ideal for diagnosis, staging
No	Yes	Yes

Melanoma specimens deserve special mention. Bread loaf vertical sectioning is the only way melanoma can be correctly staged. Horizontal or oblique sections through a melanoma excision specimen should never be contemplated. As is outlined in the melanoma chapter, a common solution to this issue is to debulk the tumor for bread loaf vertical sections and then deal with the margins separately with horizontal processing if these are needed for complete margin assessment. "Mapped excision" is a distinct term used for the management of melanoma which employs careful orientation and bread loaf processing of the entire specimen. This is discussed further in the chapter dedicated to melanoma (see Chap. 10).

Mohs Technique (*En Face* Horizontal Sectioning)

This method is usually deployed in Mohs micrographic surgery (MMS). Central to this method is that the specimen be manipulated in such a way as to allow the entire deep and radial margin to be in the same plane. Horizontal sections of this can thus be cut, allowing examination of the entire margin. The excision specimen is usually bowl-shaped, with a 45° angle or bevel (rather than the usual 90°) at the edges which allows for easier flattening. The method is outlined in **Figs. 6.9** to **6.22**.

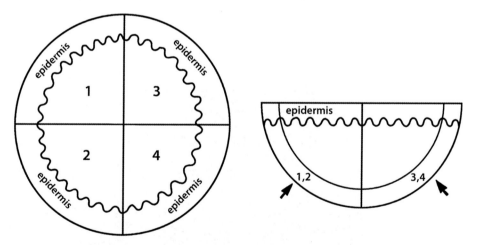

FIGURE 6.9. **The Mohs technique is the method common in MMS.** The entire margin is examined without the margin being sliced off by the pathologist. The specimen is embedded flat and microscopic sections are cut horizontally to contain the entire margin. In this illustration, the specimen has been cut into four pieces (1-4). Dividing specimens like this is essential for larger excisions that cannot fit into one tissue block. Some dermatologists prefer cutting all specimens into quadrants to aid in the processing and orientation. When no quadrants are cut and the whole specimen is processed as one, the method is sometimes referred to as "360 Mohs." On the right is the same specimen from a side perspective. These are considered "horizontal sections" as the sections run nearly parallel to the epidermis. The arrows indicate the direction which the microtome sectioning needs to follow to allow accurate representation of the entire margin. (Reproduced with permission from Rapini RP. Comparison of methods for checking surgical margins. *J Am Acad Dermatol.* 1990;23(2 Pt 1):288-294.[4])

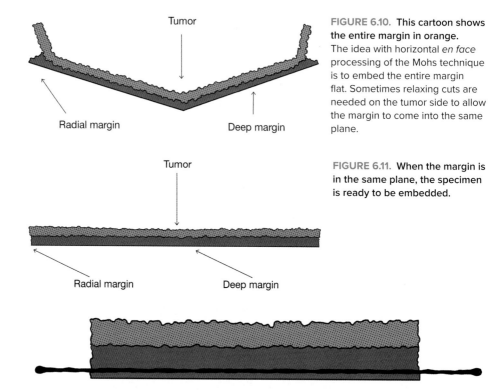

Tumor

Radial margin

Deep margin

FIGURE 6.10. **This cartoon shows the entire margin in orange.** The idea with horizontal *en face* processing of the Mohs technique is to embed the entire margin flat. Sometimes relaxing cuts are needed on the tumor side to allow the margin to come into the same plane.

Tumor

Radial margin

Deep margin

FIGURE 6.11. **When the margin is in the same plane, the specimen is ready to be embedded.**

FIGURE 6.12. Horizontal sections are cut (black line) with the microtome to allow complete assessment of the margin in one plane.

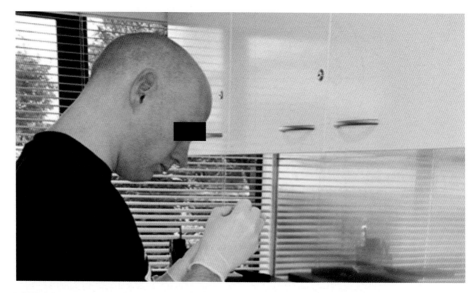

FIGURE 6.13. **The histotechnician is a key member of the team.** They must pay meticulous attention to detail to ensure the specimen is correctly labeled and handled. A key skill is the ability to manipulate the specimen so that the deep and radial margin are in the same plane for horizontal sectioning of the entire margin.

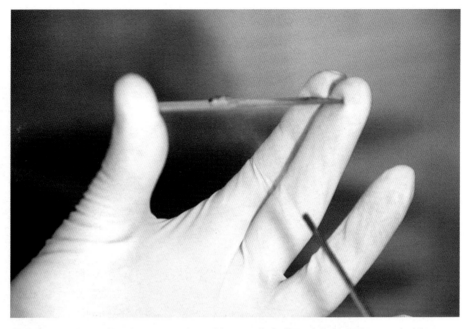

FIGURE 6.14. **Many technicians use a glass slide to assist in flattening the entire margin.** Nitrogen spray to freeze the slide helps adhere the entire deep and radial margins of the specimen to the flat surface of the slide.

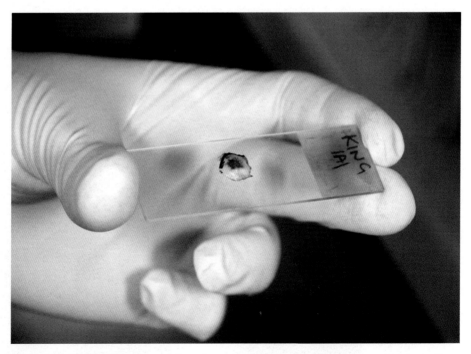

FIGURE 6.15. **The margin of the specimen is now flat against the slide.** Relaxing cuts are sometimes made on the non-margin side (the epidermis) so that the specimen can be laid flat and the entire deep and radial margin is pressed onto the perfectly flat surface of the slide.

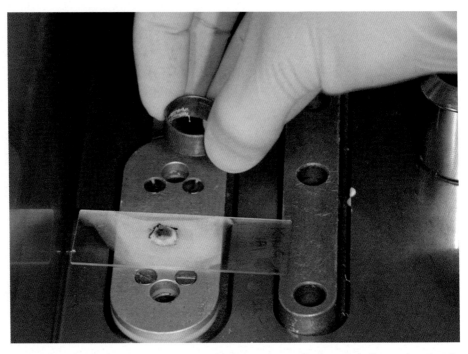

FIGURE 6.16. **There are various ways to transfer the specimen with the margin flattened against the slide to a chuck in mounting medium ready for cutting.** In the simple method shown, a metal ring is applied around the specimen.

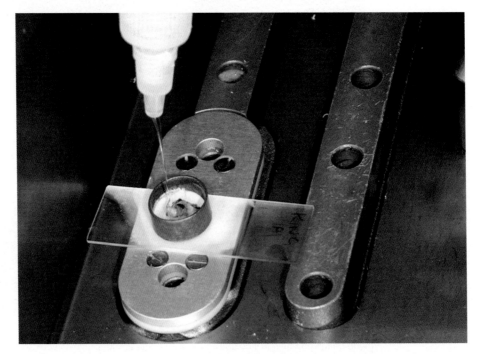

FIGURE 6.17. **The metal ring is filled with mounting medium (called OCT, optimum cutting temperature) and allowed to freeze.**

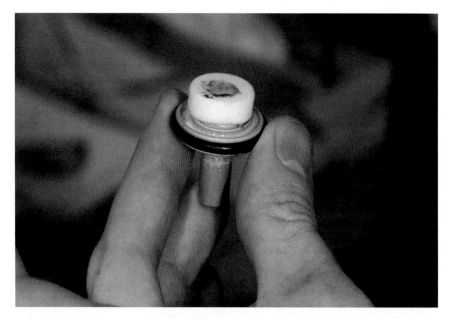

FIGURE 6.18. **The specimen frozen in mounting medium is transferred to a chuck for cryostat cutting.** It is helpful to first apply mounting medium to the chuck and then bind this to the piece of mounting material containing the flattened specimen. Otherwise, there is a risk the block of mounting medium may come off the metal chuck during the cutting of the microscopic sections. It is important that the specimen is level. Some technicians use spirit levels or other embedding devices to ensure it is completely level and ready for cutting in the cryostat.

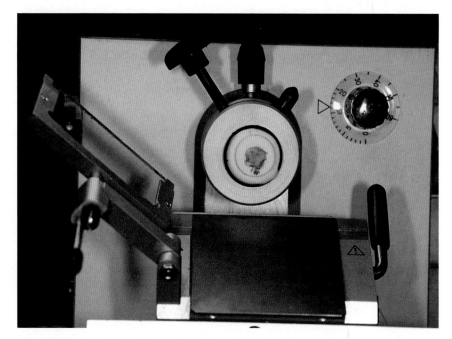

FIGURE 6.19. **The block is ready for cutting.** Given the need for complete sections and the frequent presence of fat, a stable frozen temperature is critical. Precision is crucial when a full face of the perfectly flat margin is being cut.

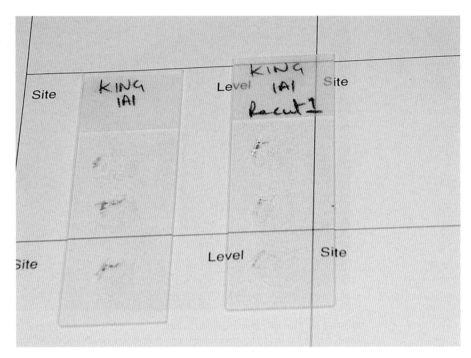

FIGURE 6.20. **The sections are laid out on glass slides.** Multiple sections are placed on each slide and multiple slides are prepared. No sections are discarded. The initial sections are usually incomplete, so cutting continues until the full margin is represented on the slides.

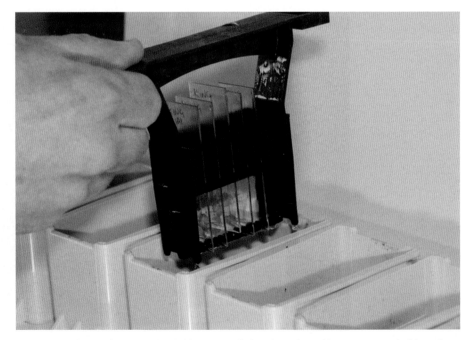

FIGURE 6.21. **The slides are stained either manually (as shown) or with an automated slide stainer.** Coverslips are applied, and the slides are ready for examination under the microscope.

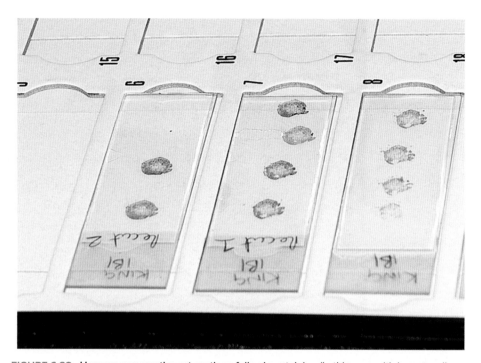

FIGURE 6.22. Here we can see the cut sections following staining (in this case with hematoxylin and eosin) and coverslipping. The initial cut sections are seen on the slide on the right. These are incomplete. Further sections are cut until the entire margin is represented on the slides (seen on the slide on the left). The pathologist must mentally reconstruct the specimen to determine whether a margin is positive. For example, if the central fat is negative for malignancy in the initial sections on the right but there is tumor present in the exact same area of central fat in complete sections on the left, the margin is still negative. Much care needs to be taken to ensure the same regions are assessed and compared between different cuts. Some practitioners prefer to call a margin positive if the tumor is within two or three cuts of the true margin.

Using a glass slide to flatten the margin allows the technician to grossly see that the deep and epidermal edges lie on the same plane without air pockets. The epidermal edge is usually unrolled on the glass side, often using minute relaxing cuts. There is a range of alternatives to this glass slide method for flattening the margin. All of them achieve the same task. These alternatives include a heat extractor, the Miami Special technique, and the Rio de Janeiro technique.[7]

Debulking the tumor with a curettage or scalpel can aid in the flattening process. Pre-excision debulking results in a thinner excision specimen which is often easier to embed. Care should be taken to avoid the carryover of tissue that can contaminate the margins.

Due to the flattening of the specimen and the cutting of the margin in a horizontal plane (horizontal to the epidermis), the reading of the slides takes some getting used to for the pathologist who is accustomed to interpreting vertical sections (**Fig. 6.23**).

This technique is almost exclusively used on fresh tissue for intraoperative frozen sections. But it can also be used in paraffin tissue. Manipulation of formalin-fixed tissue to flatten and embed in paraffin does not require a glass slide. Key features of the Mohs method are outlined in **Table 6.2**.

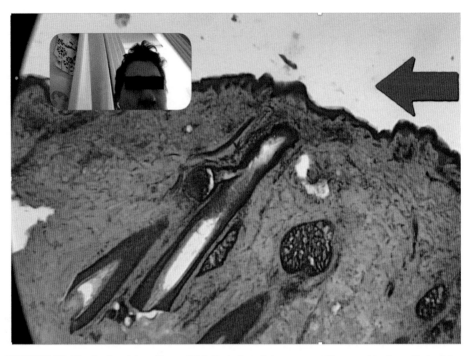

FIGURE 6.23. **The horizontal sections of this technique take some getting used to for pathologists who are accustomed to reading sections cut vertically.** With horizontal sections, the epidermis can seem thicker and the adnexal structures unusual due to tangential sectioning. Care needs to be taken not to misinterpret these features as dermal invasive tumor. This is a screenshot of a teleconference between the surgeon and pathologist who are viewing the slide together. Many teleconference applications also allow the use of arrows to facilitate communication.

TABLE 6.2 Key Features of Mohs Method		
Examines entire margin	Can measure distance to margin	Ideal for diagnosis, staging
Yes	No	No. A debulk specimen is needed.

En Face 3D Technique

This technique is basically a complete three-dimensional (3D) margin assessment without any gaps. There is considerable confusion about this technique as multiple names have been given to the same technique or techniques with minor differences. In the United States, the terms "complete circumferential peripheral and deep margin assessment" (CCPDMA) and "peripheral and deep *en face* margin assessment" (PDEMA) are commonly used.[8]

The excision specimen usually has a 90° radial angle around the edges (rather than the 45° bevel with the Mohs method). Following orientation and mapping, the surgical margins are removed by the pathologist. Approximately 3- to 5-mm-wide strips of the specimen's edges are dissected from the peripheral resection margin, divided into convenient length strips, and placed in cassettes for *en face* sections. The deep margin is also sliced off and placed in a cassette[9] (**Fig. 6.24**).

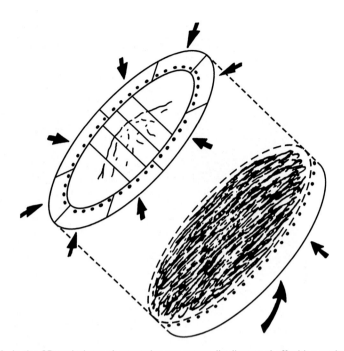

FIGURE 6.24. **In the 3D technique, the margins are generally dissected off with a scalpel and embedded *en face* for examination of the entire margin.** In the cartoon, the specimen is cut along the dotted lines. The radial margin is dissected off as thin strips of 3-5 mm, and a disk of fat is removed from the deep margin. The remaining specimen can be bread-loafed (lines across tumor) and processed in paraffin for routine diagnostic examination. The arrows indicate the direction in which the margin slices need to be cut with the cryostat or microtome so that the true margin is sectioned first. It is important that the histotechnician understand this concept. The cutting needs to start at the outermost or most peripheral side which is inked. The advantage of doing this is that minimal levels are needed and that it is easier for the pathologist to assess. The first sections cut with the cryostat or microtome represent the actual margin. Occasionally with *en face* sectioning, it may be difficult to obtain a smooth, complete slice of tissue. When this occurs, the incomplete section results in areas of the margin not being available for evaluation. If the initial section is incomplete, recuts can be obtained to gain a complete picture of the margins. (Reproduced with permission from Rapini RP. Comparison of methods for checking surgical margins. *J Am Acad Dermatol.* 1990;23(2 Pt 1):288-294.[4])

The pathologist maps any positive areas and relays this back to the surgeon (usually with a drawn diagram or map). The main specimen (now with the margins removed) can be processed in formalin and bread-loafed to allow full assessment of thickness, etc.

The "Tübinger Torte" is an *en face* 3D technique best suited for larger excisions. With this method, the specimen is inked and the entire radial margin is removed in a 2- to 3-mm-wide strip. The entire circumference is embedded *en face*, allowing examination of the entire radial margin. The deep margin is also removed and embedded flat (**Fig. 6.25**).

A slight variation of the Tübinger Torte technique is the Tübinger Muffin technique, which is more suited to smaller excisions. Longitudinal cuts are made so that the entire radial margin can be separated and carefully brought into one plane with the deep margin (**Fig. 6.26**). This is very similar to the Mohs technique, the main difference being that the excision has 90° edges rather than 45° angles around the edge.

The key features of the *en face* 3D technique are highlighted in **Tables 6.3** and **6.4**.

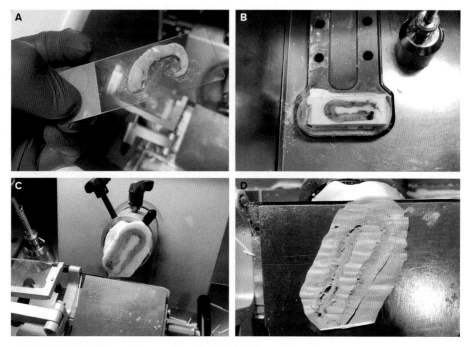

FIGURE 6.25. The Tübinger Torte and the 3D techniques are essentially equivalent. A 3-mm-wide strip of peripheral margin is removed. The deep margin is also shaved off. The entire margin is blocked (cut into a convenient size to fit on a glass slide) and embedded for frozen section. To attain a flat section of the margin, the true surgical margin is pressed against the glass slide (A) so that the margin is perfectly flat for freezing and processing (B-D). This method is carried out for the entire peripheral and deep margin.

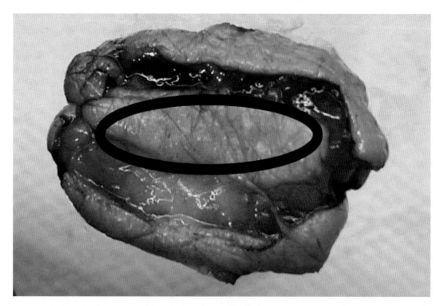

FIGURE 6.26. In the Tübinger Muffin technique, longitudinal cuts are made so that the entire radial margin can be separated and carefully brought into one plane with the deep margin. The central part of the excision (black oval) may be removed for diagnosis.

TABLE 6.3 *En Face* 3D Techniques

Advantages:
- Easier to embed than Mohs sections
- The central specimen (remaining following removal of margins) can serve as a debulk processed routinely in the laboratory.
- As the sections are not cut horizontally, interpretation is easier for pathologists who are not used to interpreting horizontal sections.

Disadvantages:
- The margin is not always in a contiguous block of tissue, which risks the margins being misinterpreted.

TABLE 6.4 Key Features of the *En Face* 3D Technique

Examines entire margin	Can measure distance to margin	Ideal for diagnosis, staging
Yes	No	Yes. The central specimen is processed vertically.

The Munich Technique

With this technique, numerous serial horizontal histologic sections are cut from the deep margin to the skin surface (**Fig. 6.27**). The horizontal sections are 6 to 10 μm thick, and between these, approximately 100 μm of tissue is discarded. This technique is not widely used as the entire margin cannot be examined despite the large number of sections requiring examination.[10] Key features of the Munich technique are highlighted in **Table 6.5**.

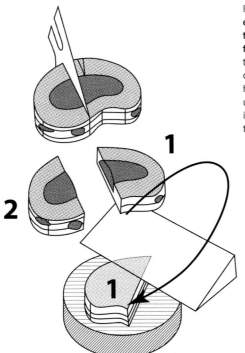

FIGURE 6.27. **In the Munich technique, the entire specimen is sectioned horizontally from the deep margin to the epidermis without flattening of the margin.** No attempt is made to manipulate the margin into one plane. In this cartoon, the specimen is divided in two and each half is processed separately. Each half is flipped upside down (arrow) and the specimen is cut horizontally all the way through the specimen from the deep margin to the surface epithelium.

TABLE 6.5 Key Features of Munich Technique

Examines entire margin	Can measure distance to margin	Ideal for diagnosis, staging
No	Yes	No

TABLE 6.6 Key Features of Perimeter Technique

Examines entire margin	Can measure distance to margin	Ideal for diagnosis, staging
No. Deep margin not examined	No	Yes

Perimeter Technique

The previous techniques allow examination of the entire radial margin but do not examine the deep margin. The square procedure, spaghetti (or linguine) technique, and the moat or perimeter technique are some names for essentially the same method of processing.

In the perimeter technique, the surgeon removes the entire radial margin in strips under local anesthetic, thereby leaving the central tumor in place until the peripheral strips have been shown to be negative for malignancy. This technique is particularly useful when radical surgery of deeper structures is needed, and delineation of radial margins is preferable before this is undertaken.[11,12] Key features of the perimeter technique are highlighted in **Table 6.6**.

A slight variation is the square technique which has been mainly applied to facial melanoma.[13] With this technique, the peripheral margin strips are removed in a square or rectangular shape. The surgeon usually removes the strips but occasionally the specimen is received as a whole and the strips can be removed by the pathologist. The squarish shape makes for an easier reconstruction and has the extra benefit of being technically easier when it comes to removing the radial margins and embedding them flat.

Peripheral Sectioning of Wedge Excisions

Given the shape of wedge excisions of the eyelid, lip, or ear, it can be much easier to remove the entire margin in slices. Examination of these *en face* ensures that the entire margin is examined (**Fig. 6.28**). Key features of the peripheral sectioning technique are highlighted in **Table 6.7**.

DEBULK CONSIDERATIONS

Debulk specimens may be important for diagnosis and staging. These are either removed by the surgeon before the wider specimen with margins is removed *or* it is the residual tissue remaining following removal of the margins by the pathologist. If the debulk is removed as a block of tissue with a scalpel, it should be processed with vertical sections as is done with the bread loaf technique. It should be serially sectioned (bread-loafed) at 3- to 4-mm intervals. If the debulk is processed in an outside laboratory, it is important to specify that no margins are required; otherwise, the pathologist will produce a report quoting the margin status and this can confuse the situation.

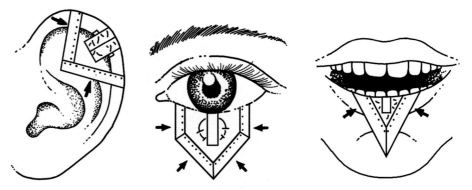

FIGURE 6.28. **For peripheral sectioning of full-thickness excisions of eyelids, ears, or lips, strips of the deep margin are removed and embedded flat so that the entire deep and radial margin is examined.** The histotechnician needs to understand that the microtome sections need to be cut in the direction of the arrows, so the real margin is examined first.

TABLE 6.7 Key Features of Peripheral Sectioning Method		
Examines 100% of margin	Can measure distance to margin	Ideal for diagnosis, staging
Yes	No	Yes. The central specimen is processed vertically, much like a debulk.

SAFETY MARGINS

Safety margins are always processed in paraffin. They are usually disks of tissue containing the whole rim of skin and deep margin taken from around the surgical defect. Sometimes only part of the margin (often just the radial margin) is submitted (**Fig. 6.28**). The margin needs to be embedded flat for sectioning to examine the entire margin as outlined in other methods (**Figs. 6.29** to **6.31**). A key advantage of the paraffin sections is that immunohistochemistry can be performed on this specimen. Though many frozen section laboratories have immunohistochemical capability, the range of antibodies is usually limited.

SPECIFIC PROCESSING ISSUES

Making histological frozen sections of skin with fat can be challenging, even with a high-quality cryostat. Key to success is to have a sufficiently frozen specimen (**Fig. 6.32**). Liquid nitrogen cooling spray offers an affordable and reliable method of helping to freeze larger specimens with abundant fat. Spray can be applied to the chuck before cutting and this is usually sufficient for obtaining full sections. Further spray can be applied in difficult cases. Artifacts can result from cooling specimens too quickly or when copious spray is applied to thin pieces of tissue (**Fig. 6.33**). Some authors have proposed cutting thicker histologic sections for adipose tissue, but this does not seem to be generally necessary.

Processing cartilage can also be challenging. Because cartilage contains sulfates which create a negative charge, the use of positively charged slides significantly helps the cartilage adhere to the slide. This adhesion to the slides can be enhanced by gently heating the slide,

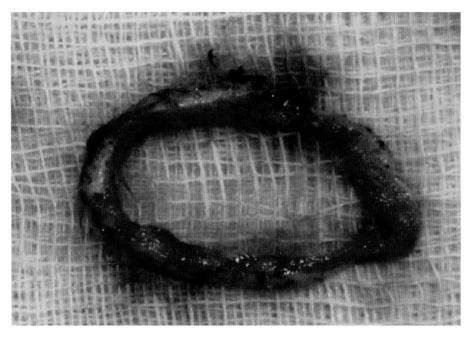

FIGURE 6.29. **The "donut" of the safety margin is sent in formalin to the laboratory for paraffin sectioning.** Often when thin strips of tissue such as this donut safety margins are placed in formalin, the tissue curls up, making embedding flat in paraffin very difficult. One option to avoid this is to pin the specimen to a board and fix it overnight before embedding in paraffin.

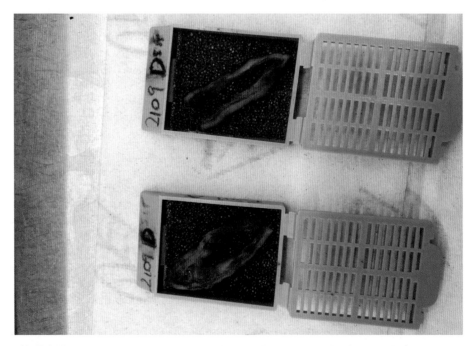

FIGURE 6.30. Another solution to prevent curling of safety margins is to place the donut directly in cassettes between foam pads after inking for orientation and before formalin fixation.

A

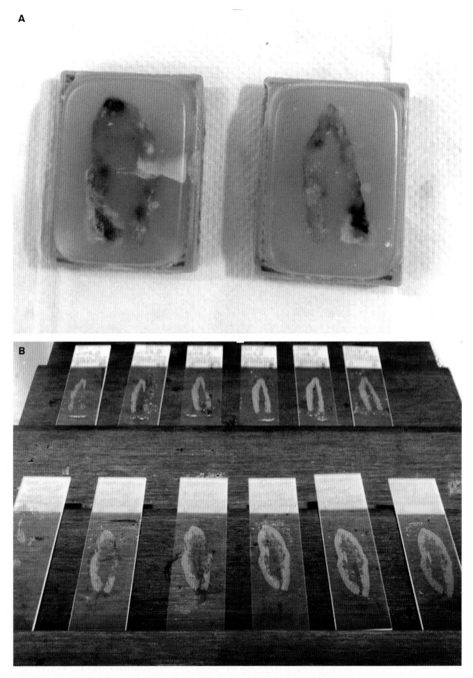

FIGURE 6.31. The safety margin is embedded in paraffin and multiple microscopic levels are cut with the microtome. If needed, immunohistochemistry can be performed on these sections.

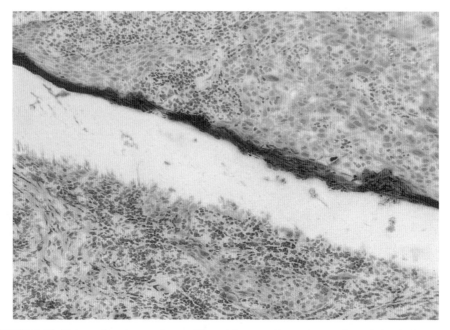

FIGURE 6.32. **This section shows a few problems.** The central areas have a linear hole which is usually the result of the cryostat being too warm and inconsistent freezing. The inflammatory cells are also smudged, which is a result of specimen manipulation/squashing. Finally, the colors look faded, which should prompt a check of the staining protocol.

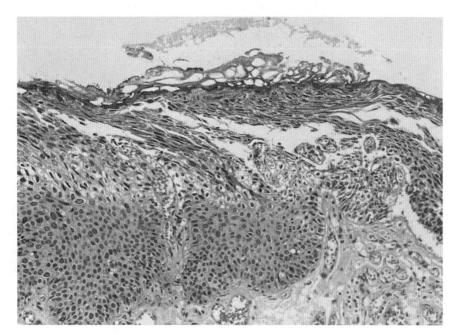

FIGURE 6.33. **This section shows marked frozen artifact change.** The top half of the epidermis shows a lack of detail and elongation of cells, making interpretation impossible in some areas. For very thin pieces of tissue, care needs to be taken when using liquid nitrogen spray.

drying the section out before fixation, and using acetone as a fixative to shorten the fixation process. Slowing the staining process will also prevent the cartilage from being washed from the slides, as will reducing the water pressure in automated stainers.[14,15]

SUMMARY

There are several methods for examining skin excision margins to achieve complete margin assessment. Familiarity with them can help in adapting in-house practices to the specimens that are received. The importance of having a trusted technical team to assist in this process cannot be overstated. Mastering the relevant skills takes an understanding of the procedures, the technical skills to process the specimen, and an understanding of laboratory protocols.

References

1. Tolkachjov SN, Brodland DG, Coldiron BM, et al. Understanding Mohs micrographic surgery: a review and practical guide for the nondermatologist. *Mayo Clin Proc.* 2017;92:1261-1271.
2. Abide JA, Nahai F, Bennett RG. The meaning of surgical margins. *Plast Reconstr Surg.* 1984;73:492-497.
3. Kimyai-Asadi A, Goldberg LH, Jih MH. Accuracy of serial transverse cross-sections in detecting residual basal cell carcinoma at the surgical margins of an elliptical excision specimen. *J Am Acad Dermatol.* 2005;53(3):469-474.
4. Rapini RP. Comparison of methods for checking surgical margins. *J Am Acad Dermatol.* 1990;23:288-294.
5. Willardson HB, Lombardo J, Raines M, et al. Predictive value of basal cell carcinoma biopsies with negative margins: a retrospective cohort study. *J Am Acad Dermatol.* 2018;79(1):42-46.
6. Alcalay J, Alkalay R. Histological evaluation of residual basal cell carcinoma after shave biopsy prior to Mohs micrographic surgery. *J Eur Acad Dermatol Venereol.* 2011;25(7):839-841.
7. Bittner GC, Cerci FB, Kubo EM, Tolkachjov SN. Mohs micrographic surgery: a review of indications, technique, outcomes, and considerations. *An Bras Dermatol.* 2021;96(3):263-277.
8. Moehrle M, Breuninger H, Röcken M. A confusing world: what to call histology of three-dimensional tumour margins? *J Eur Acad Dermatol Venereol.* 2007;21(5):591-595.
9. Danesh MJ, Menge TD, Helliwell L, Mahalingam M, Waldman A. Adherence to the National Comprehensive Cancer Network Criteria of complete circumferential peripheral and deep margin assessment in treatment of high-risk basal and squamous cell carcinoma. *Dermatol Surg.* 2020;46(12):1473-1480.
10. Boztepe G, Hohenleutner S, Landthaler M, Hohenleutner U. Munich method of micrographic surgery for basal cell carcinomas: 5-year recurrence rates with life-table analysis. *Acta Derm Venereol.* 2004;84(3):218-222.
11. Ward J, Mitsala G, Petsios M, Orlando A. Linguine technique for excision of lentigo maligna and poorly defined non-melanotic skin cancer: a case series. *JPRAS Open.* 2019;19:111-117.
12. Vance KK, Pytynia KB, Antony AK, Krunic AL. Mohs moat: peripheral cutaneous margin clearance in a collaborative approach for aggressive and deeply invasive basal cell carcinoma. *Australas J Dermatol.* 2014;55(3):198-200.
13. Johnson TM, Headington JT, Baker SR, Lowe L. Usefulness of the staged excision for lentigo maligna and lentigo maligna melanoma: the "square" procedure. *J Am Acad Dermatol.* 1997;37(5 Pt 1):758-764.
14. Shelton M. Lab pearls: making great slides. In: Gross K, Steinman HK, eds. *Mohs Surgery and Histopathology: Beyond the Fundamentals.* New York, NY: Cambridge University Press; 2009:52-56.
15. Aslam A, Aasi SZ. Frozen-section tissue processing in Mohs surgery. *Dermatol Surg.* 2019;45(Suppl 2):S57-S69.

7

Slide Preparation and Immunohistochemistry

Patrick Emanuel / Martin Cavanagh

Routine Staining
Immunohistochemistry
    Method
    Clinical and Histologic Controls
    Problems

Melanoma
Nonmelanoma Skin Cancers
DFSP
Other Tumors
Summary

ROUTINE STAINING

High-quality staining is central to the successful interpretation of pathology slides. In fact, it is probably not advisable to consider doing margin control surgery (MCS) without a well-equipped laboratory and trusted staff. Most laboratories use the hemotoxylin and eosin (HE) stain to colorize slides. This picks up the various tissue and cellular components in different ways, resulting in a highly reproducible artifact allowing assessment of the cellular and tissue morphology. Pathologists use these staining characteristics to make determinations about the features of disease they see microscopically. In a sense, it is medicine's version of *physiognomy*, the study of how someone's personality can be determined just by looking at their facial characteristics. Though it may seem superficial and far less sophisticated than an involved genetic analysis, the centuries-old method of HE staining continues to be the gold standard in diagnostic pathology.

An alternative to HE is the toluidine blue stain, a metachromatic stain which stains the mucopolysaccharides around basal cell carcinoma (BCC) a distinctive magenta color. This can be helpful in difficult and subtle cases of BCC but due to several factors—the perceived inferior cellular detail being the most pertinent—it fell out of favor and its use has largely been abandoned.

HE is composed of hematoxylin and eosin. Hematoxylin is an extract derived from the *Haematoxylum campechianum* logwood, a tree native to Mexico. This stains acidic cell components such as nucleic acids, glycosaminoglycans, and acid glycoproteins into shades of blue or purple. Eosin is an acidic dye and serves as an excellent counterstain to hematoxylin as it targets the cytoplasm of cells, specifically mitochondria, secretory granules, and collagen. It gives differing shades of pink to the cytoplasm of different types of cells and connective tissues.

TABLE 7.1 Sample Rapid Frozen Section HE Staining Method

1. Allow sections to dry on slide to ensure adhesion to slide during staining. (Slides do not dry *during* staining, only prior.)
2. Immerse in 10% neutral buffered formalin—minimum 1 minute.
3. Rinse well in tap water—four good rinses are usually advisable.
4. Gill II Hematoxylin (1 minute)
5. Rinse in tap water—four good rinses.
6. Blue in Scott's Tap Water Substitute—minimum 30 seconds
7. Rinse in tap water.
8. Alcoholic eosin (50% specially denatured ethanol and 50% water)—40 seconds
9. Rinse in tap water (not critical but saves alcohol rinses from needing constant changing due to eosin contamination).
10. Dehydrate through five changes of specially denatured alcohol (SDA)—ten dips in each of the five stations.
11. Coverslip (We use "Clearium" mountant by Surgipath which can be used straight from SDA without clearing in xylene.)

There is a range of protocols for performing the HE stain but they all have the same key steps. The first step is always slide fixation, in which chemicals or heat is used to adhere the tissue sections to the slide before staining. Frozen section laboratories typically use 10% neutral buffered formalin, alcoholic formalin, alcohol, or acetone as a fixative. If the slides are removed too quickly from the fixative, they will be inadequately dehydrated, which profoundly alters the staining quality.

Following fixation, the key steps are nuclear staining (hematoxylin), cytoplasm staining (eosin), dehydration, clearing, and coverslipping. Each one of these steps is a potential cause for morphologic distortion (**Table 7.1**).

There are two main HE methods: progressive and regressive. The main difference between them is the hematoxylin used. In the progressive method, the hematoxylin solution contains an acid which increases the binding to nuclei. Variation in color is due to the selective affinity of tissue components to hematoxylin. With the regressive method, neutral hematoxylin is used which causes an initial overstaining, and subsequent steps remove this excess stain. The progressive method is generally easier to manage and the staining is more reproducible. Some laboratories prefer the regressive method as it offers a starker contrast between the staining colors.

Automated stainers follow the same basic principles. They are almost universally used with paraffin processing and are becoming more popular in frozen section laboratories because they are seen as less time-consuming for the technical staff and decrease the risk of repetitive strain injuries. The same quality considerations as for manual staining are needed so it is important that these automated systems are staffed by people who have a comprehensive understanding of manual staining (**Tables 7.2** and **7.3**). Examples of common processing problems are shown in **Figs. 7.1** to **7.6**.

IMMUNOHISTOCHEMISTRY

Although routine HE sections are usually sufficient to assess the margins of a tumor excision, malignant cells can at times be very difficult to identify and routine interpretation can be difficult if not impossible. For example, poorly differentiated tumors may resemble inflammatory cells, and tumors may spread as single cells through tissues and be extremely difficult to see. Immunohistochemistry (IHC), with its use of a colored marker

TABLE 7.2 Practical Tips for Quality Staining

Whatever the preferred staining method, the following general best lab practices help to ensure an optimal staining result.

- It is important that the sections are of the correct thickness. Any deviation from a 5-6 μm thickness causes significant interpretation problems.
- Do not allow frozen sections to air-dry at any time during the staining procedure. Drying causes the cellular detail to blur.
- With time, the solutions become diluted or contaminated. Regular refreshing of solutions is advised.
- The solutions need to be stored away from direct sunlight, moisture, and excessive heat for best preservation.

TABLE 7.3 Common Problems with Rapid HE Staining

- Weak Hematoxylin staining: Due to inadequate staining time, excessive de-staining, weak hematoxylin due to carryover, contaminants, thin sections, and inadequate removal of alcohol or insufficient pre-rinsing with water prior to staining with hematoxylin.
- Excessive Hematoxylin staining: Due to drying of section, excessive staining times, too weak or inadequate de-staining time, thick section.
- Weak Eosin staining: Due to contaminant in the alcohol rinse, deteriorating eosin due to excessive carryover, thin sections, inadequate staining time.
- Excessive Eosin staining: Due to stronger dye solution (can be due to excessive evaporation), thick sections, excessive staining times.
- Blurry white haze under the coverslip: Due to incomplete dehydration of the section, formed by a mixture of water and the clearing agent.

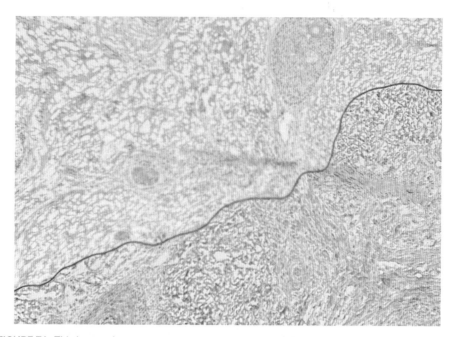

FIGURE 7.1. This image shows two common problems. On the upper aspect, you can see the insufficient hematoxylin. The nuclear detail is not vivid. This is usually due to insufficient time in the hematoxylin or diluted hematoxylin due to contamination with the other solutions. Re-staining for another 30 seconds and then washing usually fixes the problem. On the bottom aspect, the cover slip has a bubble due to insufficient mounting medium.

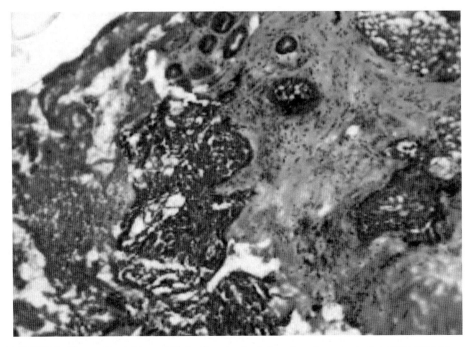

FIGURE 7.2. **The section is blurry.** This is often due to drying of sections, excessive staining times, and too weak or inadequate de-staining time.

(chromogen) that is visible with a light microscope, allows for a more confident assessment when distinguishing tumor from surrounding cells.

IHC has been an integral part of diagnostic surgical pathology for decades. Both frozen tissue and tissue embedded in paraffin are suitable for processing. Paraffin IHC takes more time, as steps are needed to undo the effect of formaldehyde fixation which results in protein cross-linking (methylene bridges) and restricted antigen-antibody binding. To remedy this difficulty, antigen retrieval methods are used which break the methylene bridges and enhance antibody binding.

Method
Though there are various ways of performing IHC, most laboratories use what is known as the *indirect* method. Briefly, this involves incubating the tissue with a primary antibody (which binds to the antigen in question), then a secondary antibody with a peroxidase label is added to amplify the signal. A chromogen is then added which, in the presence of the peroxidase-labeled antibody, will form an insoluble colored product. Commonly used chromogens include 3,3'-diaminobenzidine tetrachloride, which forms a brown product, or 3-amino-9-ethylcarbazole, which forms a red product (**Fig. 7.7**).

A modification of this technique is the *direct* method. In the direct method, no secondary antibody is needed as the label is present on the primary antibody. As there is no amplification with the secondary antibody, the signal is weaker. The basic steps are outlined in **Table 7.4**.

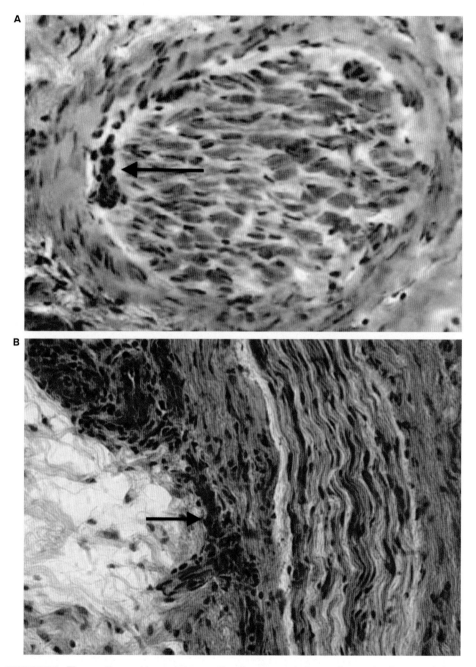

FIGURE 7.3. The small vessel (arrow) surrounding the nerve mimics carcinoma due to excessive hematoxylin staining. This may be caused by drying of the section, excessive staining times, or inadequate de-staining time.

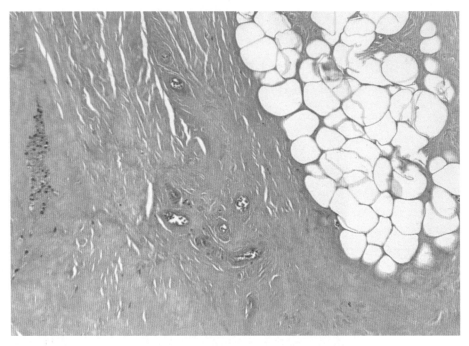

FIGURE 7.4. Thick sections pick up too much stain and the cellular detail is lost.

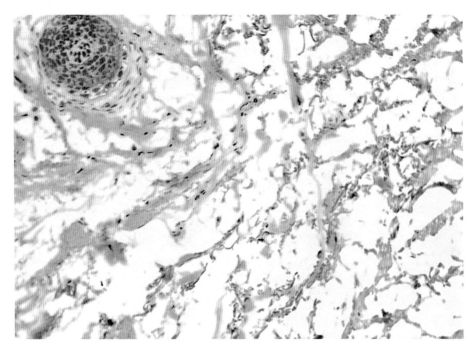

FIGURE 7.5. When the cryostat blade is slightly dull, gaps appear in the sections.

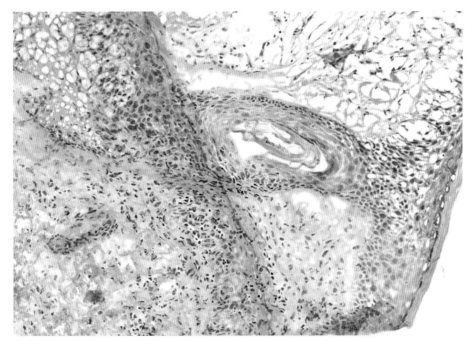

FIGURE 7.6. **Section folding commonly occurs if the processing is rushed and attention is not given to ensure the section is laid flat on the slide.** This folding may cause the pathology to be uninterpretable.

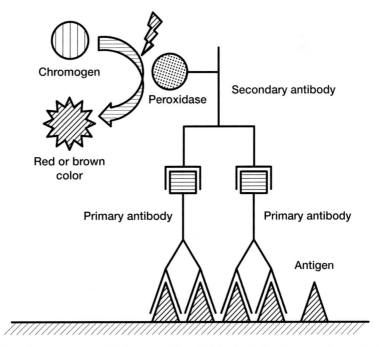

FIGURE 7.7. **Indirect method of IHC.** The peroxidase (Px) is attached to the secondary antibody which is specific to the primary antibody.

TABLE 7.4 Basic Steps (Indirect Method)

1. Prepare tissue sections and undertake antigen retrieval
2. Block with serum (same species as secondary antibody, reduces antibody binding to background cells)
3. Add primary antibody
4. Wash
5. Add secondary antibody which is already conjugated with an enzyme (peroxidase)
6. Wash
7. Add chromogen
8. Wash
9. Counterstain (e.g., hematoxylin)
10. Mount slide and interpret with microscope

Modifications can be made in-house to optimize the procedure and reduce the time required. The multitude of publications outlining ever-shorter protocols demonstrates the wide variation possible with individual IHC stains.[3,4] Examples of common modifications include increasing the concentration of the antibody, reducing blocking steps, and using secondary antibodies with enhanced detection systems (e.g., secondary antibodies may come with already bound spherical polymer and more peroxidase enzymes). When dealing with paraffin tissue, antigen retrieval methods such as heating and applying heavy metal–containing solutions or citrate buffers are commonly used to enhance IHC.

Clinical and Histologic Controls

For each clinical case, the IHC reagents are subject to controls to maximize the accuracy of IHC reagents. It is up to the testing laboratory to establish these quality control procedures. Histologically, positive and negative antibody controls confirm the IHC reagent performance for every IHC run. A central debulk specimen of the tumor can serve as a control. Alternatively, native benign cells can also serve as internal controls such as normal melanocytes in cases of melanoma, or epithelial structures (hairs, epidermis) in carcinoma cases. Clinical controls have become popular in melanoma surgery. A biopsy of nonlesional skin is stained with a melanocytic IHC marker to assess the normal background density of melanocytes.

Problems

The manufacturers of the IHC reagents provide detailed guidelines regarding the concentration and volumes of reagents and timing of the steps. Even so, the actual results seen in individual laboratories show considerable variation and it usually takes several trials to introduce a new antibody into a laboratory.

Aside from proving protocols work in-house, paying proper attention to high-quality slide preparation is key to high-quality IHC. Sections must be thin enough (4 μm) to allow adequate diffusion and binding of the antibodies. Charged slides facilitate the bonding of the section and minimize the loss of parts of sections during processing. Finally, sections need to be laid flat by the histotechnician without gaps, holes, or folds. This is particularly difficult for frozen section preparation of larger specimens with large amounts of adipose tissue.[1]

Modifications to protocols to decrease time require special attention to quality, and thus controls are vitally important. For example, reducing the time of the blocking agent or washing steps may shorten the procedure but the consequence may be higher background nonspecific staining.[2]

TABLE 7.5 Melanoma IHC

Antibody	Staining	Redeeming Qualities	Problems
S100	Nuclear and cytoplasmic	Highly sensitive, including in unusual and desmoplastic melanoma	Less specific (stains intraepidermal Langerhans cells, nerves, normal melanocytes, adipose tissue)
Melan-A	Cytoplasmic	Highly sensitive and specific. Easy-to-use kits available for frozen section processing	Negative in desmoplastic melanoma. Keratinocytes may stain positively, particularly in lichenoid reactions. Stains normal melanocytes
HMB-45	Cytoplasmic	Highly specific	Negative in a percentage of melanoma, desmoplastic melanoma. Positive in normal melanocytes
Sox-10	Nuclear	Highly sensitive. Nuclear staining easier to interpret	Positive in nerves, fat, myoepithelial cells, and normal melanocytes
PRAME	Nuclear	Distinguishes melanoma from benign melanocytic lesions	Literature lacking its utility in assessing margins on sun-damaged skin

Melanoma

A variety of antibodies has been used in assessing surgical margins in excision of melanoma. These have been summarized in **Table 7.5**. IHC has particular use in distinguishing populations of melanocytes within freeze artifact, spongiosis, and keratinocytic atypia.

In the context of MCS, a highly sensitive, specific stain is needed. HMB-45 is a very specific stain for melanocytes but not as sensitive. S100 is highly sensitive but is less specific, particularly in the epidermis where it stains native Langerhans cells. These markers have fallen out of favor in recent years due to the introduction of alternatives.

Melan-A (Mart 1) has become the most widely used antibody in MCS for melanoma as it is both highly sensitive and specific. Protocols have been developed to allow rapid processing and evaluation intraoperatively on frozen section material, and margins are sometimes assessed with Melan-A in paraffin with a rapid method to help delineate margins. Normal melanocytes can serve as an internal control. Distribution and density of melanocytes are key to distinguishing melanoma from normal melanocytes. Nesting, increased density, melanocytes in the upper levels of the epidermis (pagetoid spread) or down adnexal structures, and enlargement are features seen in melanoma, but none are diagnostic. Experience is necessary when interpreting Melan-A to avoid overestimating the number of true melanocytes. Dendritic processes from melanocytes wrapped around keratinocytes may lead to a false-positive staining result. Keratinocytes on sun-damaged skin and within a lichenoid infiltrate may stain positively with Melan-A, which presents a potential pitfall. Finally, because the stain is positive in the cytoplasm, interpretation can be difficult when there are numerous pigment-laden macrophages. Given its relatively widespread use, it is not surprising that there is a large body of literature outlining innovations in staining protocols which decrease time demand while maintaining quality. Protocols have reported processing times as short as 19 minutes, with results analogous to those seen with paraffin processing.[4]

Sox-10 is a clean nuclear stain, so interpretation may be easier than with Melan-A, especially in cases with inflammation and dermal melanophages obscuring the lesion. It was thought to be useful in distinguishing desmoplastic melanoma from dermal scar, but Sox-10 does show some staining in scars, so care needs to be taken in this context.

PReferentially expressed Antigen in Melanoma (PRAME) has gained a great deal of attention recently in the dermatopathology literature. Nuclear staining is seen in the majority of melanomas and is uncommon in benign melanocytes. In the delineation of margins, it was shown to correlate well with the findings on HE. It could be helpful in the delineation of margins in patients with significant sun damage and background melanocytic hyperplasia. However, there is limited literature to date regarding the utility of PRAME in the margin control literature.

Critical to the interpretation of Melan-A and the other markers is an understanding of the normal range of melanocytic density. Higher-than-normal numbers of melanocytes at the margin of a melanoma excision suggest melanoma, but defining what an *increased* number of melanocytes actually is has proved difficult. This is discussed in greater detail in the chapter dedicated to melanoma. Nonmalignant sun-damaged skin can have up to 15 melanocytes per high-power field and show confluence of up to nine adjacent melanocytes as well as extension of melanocytes along hair follicles. A greater number than this would be a worrisome finding. Nesting and significant spread into the upper layers of the epidermis (pagetoid spread) is not usually observed in normal sun-exposed skin and suggests melanoma.

Nonmelanoma Skin Cancers

A variety of stains have been used in the context of margin control in BCC and SCC (**Table 7.6**). These stains are helpful in finding subtle perineural carcinoma and subtle tumors with a single-cell infiltrative pattern, as well as in cases where the tumor is masked by a dense lymphocytic response. AE1/AE3 is a commercially available stain useful for the identification of carcinoma. AE1/AE3 is a cocktail of various cytokeratin antibodies and is helpful in capturing a broad range of keratinocytic differentiation including BCC and the various degrees of differentiation in SCC.

One issue with a broad-spectrum cytokeratin is that it lacks specificity in finding carcinoma. p63, and more recently p40, are clean nuclear stains which have been applied to a variety of tumors in surgical pathology. These are extremely sensitive in staining carcinoma and can be helpful in highlighting subtle residual carcinoma at surgical margins and around nerves (**Fig. 7.8**). CK5/6 is a high-molecular-weight keratin, it is also used widely in skin carcinomas. It has less utility in the margin control context since a significant percentage of SCC and BCC are negative.

DFSP

Because distinguishing DFSP from scar tissue and normal fibroblasts can be challenging, IHC staining with CD34 can assist in delineating the tumor either intraoperatively with frozen sections or in paraffin. While CD34 is very sensitive and an excellent marker for

TABLE 7.6 Carcinoma IHC

Antibody	Staining	Advantage	Disadvantage
AE1/AE3	Cytoplasmic	Sensitive	Not specific. Stains practically all epithelial cells and carcinomas. Positive in some sarcomas
CK5/6	Cytoplasmic	Specific	Some SCC and BCC are negative
p63/p40	Nuclear	Sensitive, nuclear stain	Positive in some sarcoma

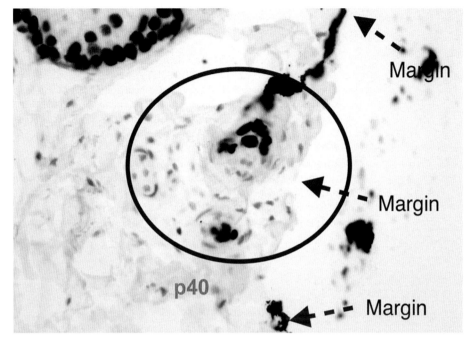

FIGURE 7.8. **IHC with p40 highlights subtle perineural infiltration at the nerve.** (Courtesy of Dr. John Snow, Wellington, New Zealand.)

DFSP, it needs to be remembered that CD34 is found in multiple cell types, including hematopoietic stem cells, endothelium, and dendritic cells of the dermal, periadnexal, and endoneuronal varieties. In addition, variable expression of CD34 may be seen in nodular areas of DFSP or areas with fibrosarcomatous differentiation. When applying CD34 in the MCS context, awareness of its limitations and the knowledge gained by experience are crucial.[5,6]

Other Tumors

IHC can be applied to a wide range of other tumors in which the HE stain is difficult to interpret. Specific examples include CK7 or CEA for extramammary Paget disease, CK20 for Merkel cell carcinoma, and CD31 in angiosarcoma. It is important that the tumor is proven to be positive with the same IHC antibody protocol being used in MCS. The best way of ensuring this is by using tumoral tissue removed during MCS (such as from the central debulk specimen) as an internal control.

SUMMARY

HE staining is key to histopathologic interpretation and requires a thorough understanding of staining principles. There are numerous potential sources of error, and an understanding of the staining steps is crucial when considering how to fix these. IHC provides valuable diagnostic and margin assessment assistance. Similar to HE staining, a good understanding of IHC is key to high-quality staining and accurate interpretation.

References

1. Miller CJ, Sobanko JF, Zhu X, et al. Special stains in Mohs surgery. *Dermatol Clin.* 2011;29:273-286.
2. El Tal AK, Abrou AE, Stiff MA, Mehregan DA. Immunostaining in Mohs micrographic surgery: a review. *Dermatol Surg.* 2010;36(3):275-290.
3. Cherpelis BS, Moore R, Ladd S, et al. Comparison of MART-1 frozen sections to permanent sections using a rapid 19-minute protocol. *Dermatol Surg.* 2009;35(2):207-213.
4. Cherpelis BS, Turner L, Ladd S, et al. Innovative 19-minute rapid cytokeratin immunostaining of non-melanoma skin cancer in Mohs micrographic surgery. *Dermatol Surg.* 2009;35(7):1050-1056.
5. Veronese F, Boggio P, Tiberio R, et al. Wide local excision vs. Mohs Tübingen technique in the treatment of dermatofibrosarcoma protuberans: a two-centre retrospective study and literature review. *J Eur Acad Dermatol Venereol.* 2017;31:2069-2076.
6. Massey RA, Tok J, Strippoli BA, Szabolcs MJ, Silvers DN, Eliezri YD. A comparison of frozen and paraffin sections in dermatofibrosarcoma protuberans. *Dermatol Surg.* 1998;24(9):995-998.

SECTION III
Applications for Cutaneous Malignancy

8

Basal Cell Carcinoma

Patrick Emanuel / Mark Izzard

Evidence
Examination
Biopsy
Basic Histopathology
Risk Stratification
  Histopathology
    Low-Risk BCC, Histology
High-Risk BCC, Histology
Perineural Invasion and Depth of Invasion
Site
Primary Versus Recurrence
Patient Factors
Histopathology Pitfalls
Summary

Though basal cell carcinoma (BCC) is the most common malignancy in the world, its incidence is not recorded in most cancer registries and published figures are probably underestimated. Estimated incidence varies within geographical and ethnic contexts, reaching almost epidemic proportions in some countries. Exposure to UV radiation is a key risk factor, particularly at a young age. The world is increasingly becoming "sun smart," but there is still a huge lag phase to work through. Alongside an increasing incidence, there are several anatomic subsites in which BCC is becoming increasingly prevalent, such as the pinna, the nose, the upper lip, and the medial eyelid.

BCC typically spreads slowly and in a predictable manner, and usually does not exhibit satellitosis. Why does BCC behave in such a predictable clinical fashion? One way of thinking about this curiosity is to consider the environmental interplay between cancer cells, immune responses, and other local factors as a *complex nonlinear system*. In this system, a degree of chaos (unpredictability) may arise in which minute changes within the system result in instability and unpredictable changes in the tumor's behavior. This chaos may manifest as a surprisingly aggressive outcome such as the occurrence of metastasis in tumors staged to be low risk. Melanoma and breast cancer are two good examples of tumors which are prone to producing chaotic conditions and clinical unpredictability. The conditions which create these less-than-desirable conditions are remarkably rare with BCC, so complete surgical excision is almost invariably curative.

Given this predictability, BCC is an excellent tumor for dealing with via margin control surgery (MCS) and represents the mainstay of malignancy in the surgical population of a margin control surgeon. The typical presentation is a small manageable tumor, but some cases present quite late and can be large or even massive by the time a patient seeks further assessment. Indications for MCS for BCC can be found in Chap. 4.

EVIDENCE

Perhaps surprisingly, there have only been a few prospective studies comparing the efficacy of MCS with wide local excision (WLE) processing. In one large prospective study, nonrecurrent tumors ($n = 397$) and recurrent tumors ($n = 201$) were examined in two arms: One treated with excision and WLE processing, and the other treated with MCS. After 10 years of follow-up, a significantly higher local recurrence rate was observed in the group treated with WLE processing. A similarly designed study of 553 BCC showed twice as many excisions had true negative surgical margins in the MCS arm.[1-3] Another randomized control study examined 408 facial BCCs and showed a 10-year cumulative probability of recurrence of 4.4% after MCS and 12.2% after WLE processing. For recurrent BCC, cumulative 10-year recurrence probabilities were 3.9% and 13.5% for MCS and WLE processing, respectively.[4]

EXAMINATION

BCC presents in a variety of clinical forms, from subtle flat patches to obvious nodules and sometimes large masses. Clinical diagnosis of skin lesions is a skill that is best acquired through reinforcement and it is good practice to become familiar with the procedure of self-auditing, recording the preoperative diagnosis, and comparing it with the final pathologic diagnosis. The many faces of BCC may be mistaken for any number of lesions: Simple nevi, seborrheic keratosis, dermatitis, and squamous cell carcinoma (SCC) are common differentials.

There are some features of presentation that BCCs often have in common:
- Slow growth
- Contact bleeding or failure to heal
- Appearance is often described as "pearly," but this is a poor descriptor. They have a translucent quality with the proliferation of vessels in a telangiectatic manner, similar to freshly filleted fish rather than the opacity of a pearl. Bluish-pink color is common in superficial lesions whereas nodular lesions are often paler.

Nodular BCC tends to grow in a regular fashion. On examination with the naked eye and dermatoscope (**Fig. 8.1**), they often have the following:
- A radial growth pattern that is regular
- Raised or rolled edges at the advancing tumor front with a sunken, sometimes ulcerated center as they grow
- Usually well-circumscribed borders
- Arborizing vessels (a central stem vessel with multiple branches ending in capillaries like a tree, usually bright red and well defined). Although this nonspecific finding presents in many skin malignancies, it helps aid diagnosis in combination with other features.

Superficial BCC can be trickier to spot (**Fig. 8.2**). It is often flat and can be scaly and irregular in shape. Although it can occur on the face, it is more often seen on the trunk. It can have multiple small erosions on the background of an unremarkable pale pink or reddish lesion.

Infiltrating BCC can also be challenging to spot. It may be dismissed by a patient as a scar from an old injury as it often presents with an indistinct whitish irregular area that resembles a scar. It can infiltrate nerves and muscles and is usually much more invasive and extensive than initially suspected (**Fig. 8.3**).

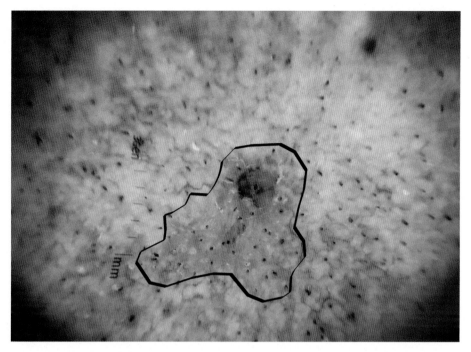

FIGURE 8.1. Dermatoscopic examination is an integral part of the assessment for diagnosis and delimitation of the extent of the lesion. This is a valuable step in planning the first level of excision.

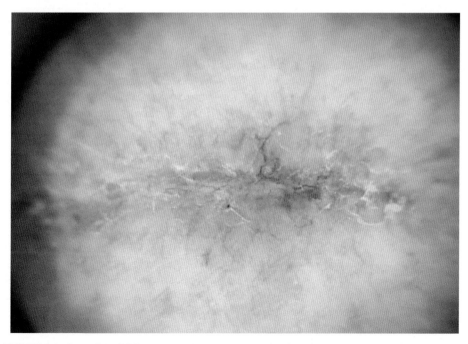

FIGURE 8.2. Superficial BCC may be misinterpreted as an eczematous or other inflammatory process for years before the diagnosis is made. Dermatoscopic examination can be extremely helpful. Arborizing vessels, telangiectasia, and focal ulceration can be suggestive.

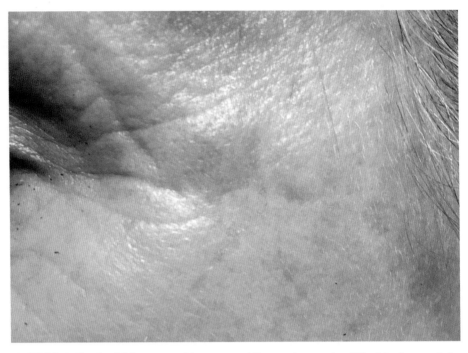

FIGURE 8.3. **Infiltrative BCC can resemble a scar and the margins may be difficult to discern clinically.** MCS is ideal for these tumors to ensure complete removal.

Massive tumors need special consideration in relation to the possible invasion of deep structures such as bone, named nerves, or the parotid gland. Multidisciplinary input on whether to include a preoperative radiologic assessment and a radiation oncology opinion may be helpful in these neglected cases. As mentioned, metastasis is an extremely uncommon event in BCC but when it does occur, the primary tumor is generally very large (>5 cm), so in these cases of massive primaries, preoperative radiologic studies may also be warranted to rule out metastasis.

Usually, a narrow rim of 1 to 2 mm is drawn with a pen around the identified extent of the BCC for the excision of the first level. Proficiency in dermatoscopy or confocal microscopy can assist this process.

BIOPSY

Critical to surgical excision is diagnosing the BCC correctly. Many surgeons will declare, "I know a BCC when I see one," believing that a BCC merely requires simple excision and that a biopsy is not necessary. A central philosophy of MCS and this book is to avoid *guesswork*. All investigations are done with clear intent in mind, and the biopsy is no different. Key information gleaned from the biopsy includes the histologic subtype of BCC, the presence of perineural invasion, and the depth of invasion. The reporting methods used by pathologists vary widely so it is worth communicating both the reasons for the biopsy and the desired information.

For smaller, more superficial lesions, a shave biopsy is a reliable way to make the diagnosis. One of the main advantages of this technique is that there is no suture to be removed and if the diagnosis turns out to be nonmalignant, the cosmetic outcome is often superior to that of a punch biopsy.

Deeper, larger lesions may not be well represented with a superficial shave biopsy. In these cases, a punch biopsy or incisional biopsy is preferred to increase the chances of an accurate diagnosis and tumor subtyping.

BASIC HISTOPATHOLOGY

The most obvious microscopic feature of BCC is that it is a basaloid epithelial tumor. (**Figs. 8.4** to **8.13**).

RISK STRATIFICATION

Knowing the histopathologic growth pattern prior to excision and combining this with the anatomic site and patient factors can guide the surgeon as to the likely size, depth, and chance of a positive margin. An in-house grading and planning system can help schedule patients for the appropriate duration of surgery.

Histopathology

When considering the histopathology, the most practical approach to stratifying risk is to adopt a two-tier histopathology system: high risk and low risk. An easy-to-apply and

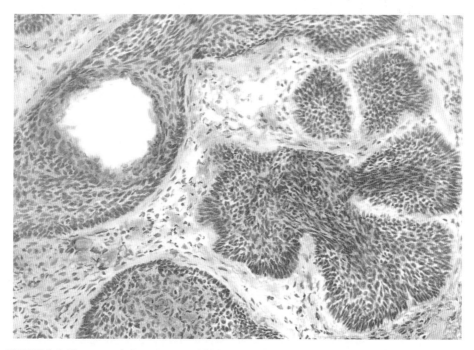

FIGURE 8.4. The most obvious feature of BCC is that it is a basaloid epithelial tumor. Most of the tumor cells are square-shaped, but the cells on the edge of the nests are more oval-shaped and line up in a row, i.e., a palisading pattern. The peritumoral stroma is hypocellular and rich in hyaluronic acid and other neutral mucins.

TABLE 8.1 Classification of BCC

Who Terminology	Terminology Used in Ontrac Trial
Infiltrative BCC	High-risk BCC, infiltrative pattern
Micronodular BCC	High-risk BCC, micronodular pattern
Sclerosing/Morpheaform BCC	High-risk BCC, infiltrative pattern with sclerotic stroma
Nodular BCC	Low-risk BCC, nodular pattern
Superficial BCC	Low-risk BCC, superficial pattern

logical system was adopted for the ONTRAC study[5] which also aligns with the National Comprehensive Cancer Network (NCCN) (**Table 8.1**). High-risk patterns have infiltrative borders histologically, often correlating to an invasive clinical presentation. Given that the biopsy represents only a fraction of the entire lesion, sometimes an aggressive histology may only come to light intraoperatively.

LOW-RISK BCC, HISTOLOGY

Nodular BCC Tumors with a predominance (i.e., >50%) of larger nodules (>0.15-mm diameter) are classified as nodular BCC. A common pitfall is to misclassify a tumor with a small area of micronodules as a micronodular BCC (**Fig. 8.5**).

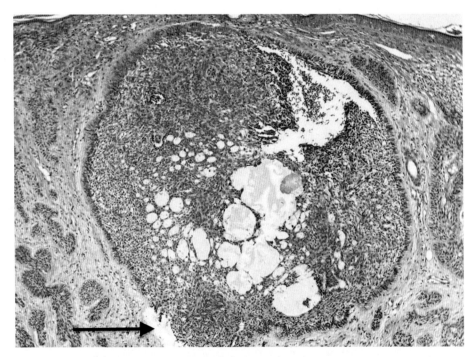

FIGURE 8.5. Nodular BCC is composed predominantly of large (>0.15 mm) nodules of tumor cells. Mucin contracts upon fixation and processing, resulting in artifactual separation of the tumor nests from the surrounding stroma. This retraction artifact (arrow) is a helpful diagnostic feature. Note that there are some small tumor nodules but given the predominant pattern has large nodules (>50%), this is best classified histopathologically as a low-risk BCC.

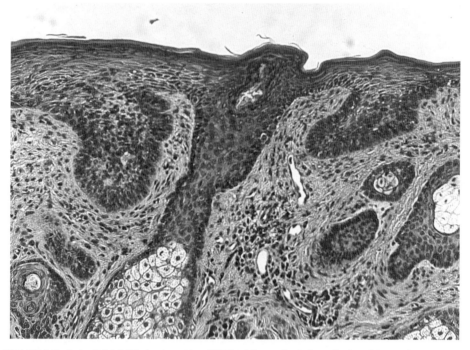

FIGURE 8.6. Superficial BCC shows nests of BCC arising as buds from the basal layer of the epidermis. These nests remain confined to the papillary dermis.

Superficial BCC This variant buds off the basal epidermis and is confined to the papillary dermis. No dermal nodules of tumor are seen (**Fig. 8.6**).

HIGH-RISK BCC, HISTOLOGY

Micronodular BCC This variant is composed predominantly (i.e., >50%) of small discrete tumor nodules (<0.15 mm in diameter). It usually has an irregular/tentacular architecture and an infiltrative deep or peripheral edge (an irregular interface at the deep or peripheral margins of the tumor with its adjacent stroma) (**Fig. 8.7**).

Infiltrative BCC This variant shows small irregular/jagged nests of tumor cells with an irregular/tentacular infiltrative/permeating pattern of invasion at the invasive tumor front (**Fig. 8.8**). The morpheic subtype is an infiltrative BCC with a dense fibrous/keloidal-like stroma.

Other Subtypes Approximately 62 other BCC subtypes have been reported in the literature. The WHO Classification of Skin Tumors defines 13 main BCC variants with an additional seven "miscellaneous" variants. Distinguishing all these types is interesting but probably not practical and there is considerable interobserver subjectivity. Tellingly, the diagnosis of BCC subtypes based upon a review of 100 BCCs by six dermatopathologists showed poor agreement (κ 0.301, $p < 0.001$).[6]

Despite this subjectivity, there are three less-common subtypes which are quite easy to define, relevant to MCS, and appear in risk category tables:

1. Sarcomatoid (**Fig. 8.9**)
2. Pinkus type (**Fig. 8.10**)
3. Basosquamous carcinoma (or Metatypical BCC) (**Fig. 8.11**)

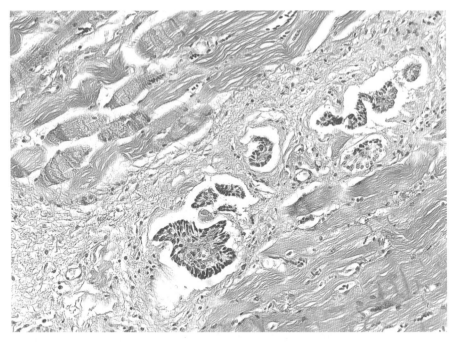

FIGURE 8.7. **Micronodular BCC is considered a high-risk tumor by the NCCN.** In this field, the tumor is composed of small nests of tumor (0.15 mm or less) at the infiltrating border. Many BCCs have small areas with this micronodular histology, but the tumor should not be classified as micronodular unless this is the predominant pattern, particularly at the invading edge.

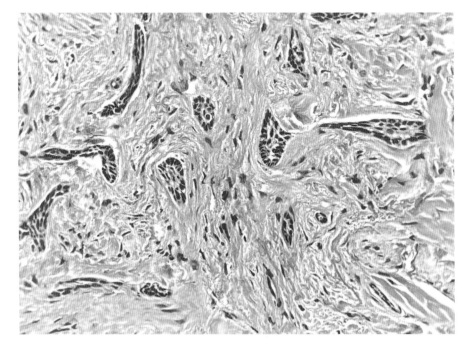

FIGURE 8.8. **BCC is seen invading the dermis with an infiltrative growth pattern of strands and single cells.** Morpheaform and sclerosing BCCs show the same pattern, but in addition, elicit a fibrotic response.

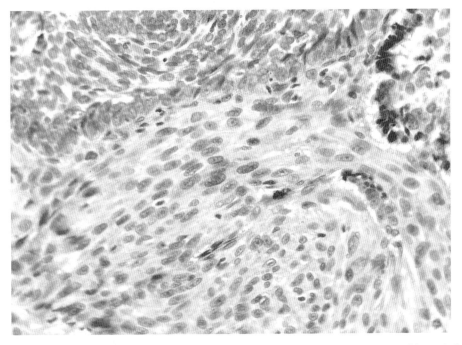

FIGURE 8.9. **In sarcomatoid BCC, regular BCC is seen dedifferentiating into a sarcomatoid morphology, sometimes as spindled cells as seen here.** Regular BCC (upper aspect) is seen directly adjacent to the sarcomatoid component. These are regarded as high-risk BCCs.

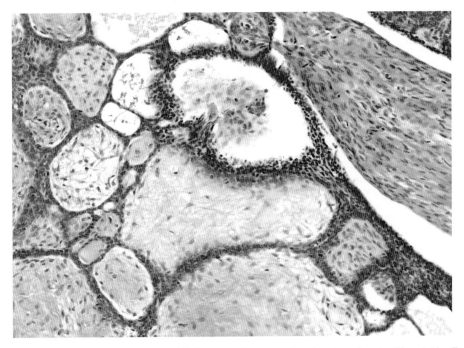

FIGURE 8.10. **BCC fibroepithelioma of Pinkus type.** Anastomosing strands and cords of basaloid cells connected to the epidermis. These are regarded as low-risk BCCs.

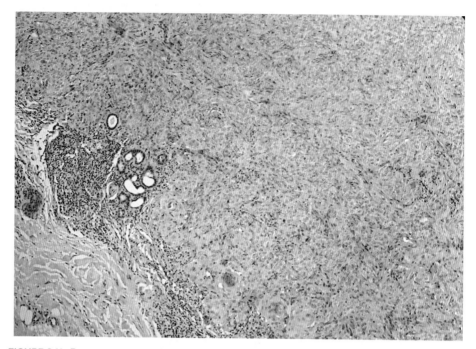

FIGURE 8.11. Basosquamous carcinoma shows areas indistinguishable from SCC intermixed with BCC. An infiltrative pattern is generally a feature. Small areas of squamous differentiation within low-risk BCC should not be considered a basosquamous carcinoma.

Basosquamous carcinomas are regarded as high risk, but this term is overused as the definition is quite loose. Low-grade regular nodular BCCs may have areas of squamous differentiation but these should not be considered basosquamous carcinomas. The term "basosquamous" should be reserved for infiltrative BCCs which have areas that resemble invasive SCCs.

Perineural Invasion and Depth of Invasion

MCS is the only precise way of localizing, tracking, and clearing perineural invasion in real time. Prior knowledge of perineural invasion, and classification into large or small nerves, is ideal; forewarned is forearmed. Not infrequently, these features are not evident in biopsy specimens and only come to light during MCS. For staging purposes with the AJCC, nerve invasion is considered significant if the nerve measures 0.1 mm or greater in the dermis or else involves any nerve in the subcutis. Numbness or a tingling sensation can be key clinical features to suggest perineural invasion (**Figs. 8.12** and **8.13**).

For advanced cases involving deep structures such as bone or the parotid gland, or in which nerves are extensively involved, a combined approach is sometimes used. The entire radial skin margins are processed intraoperatively and the deeper excision is sent for paraffin examination if frozen section examination is not feasible.

Site

It is useful to stratify BCC based on anatomic location as well. This is useful for surgical planning, time management, and managing patient expectations and outcomes. For example, infiltrating BCC with perineural invasion on the nose will require much more surgical

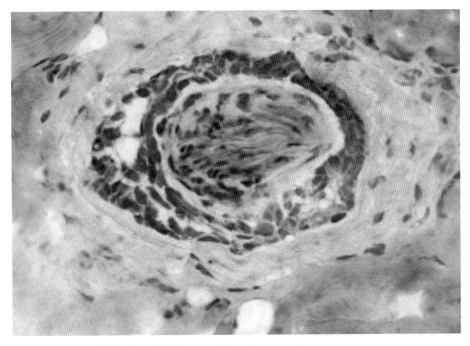

FIGURE 8.12. **Nerve infiltration of BCC encountered intraoperatively.**

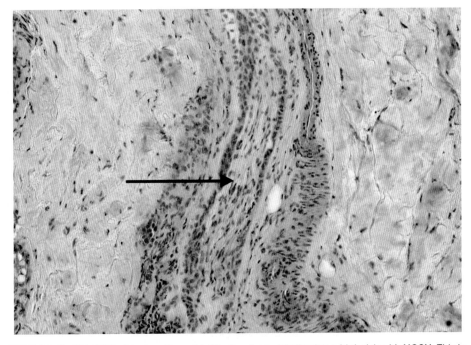

FIGURE 8.13. **This BCC shows perineural infiltration (arrow) indicating a high risk with NCCN.** This is a photo from intraoperative margin assessment during MCS.

time as well as the possibility of multiple levels and a complex reconstruction when compared with a nodular BCC in the same location.

Primary Versus Recurrence

Unfortunately, recurrent lesions are not rare in populations with a high incidence of BCC, particularly if previous surgical excisions have not been managed with MCS. Recurrent BCC can often be multifocal and may require extensive mapping and long procedures to clear. This is particularly the case if a rotation flap has been employed previously, in which case it is difficult to identify areas of multifocal recurrence. Generally, the entire scar of the previous excision will be encompassed in the final defect.

Patient Factors

The decision to proceed with surgery is always taken with the patient in mind, and it is a balancing act between morbidity and mortality. Even the smallest lesion can cause significant patient distress and morbidity. No patient wants surgery, and all patients wish to remain as unchanged as possible after the ordeal. With this in mind, surgical planning is paramount as is discussion encompassing techniques, the surgical procedure, and likely outcomes, including showing patients before-and-after photos.

Very large lesions and lesions arising in both immunosuppressed patients, as well as patients with a history of numerous high-risk carcinomas, will also need special consideration. In practice, the patient cares little for surgical techniques and just wants to look normal again after the procedure and, importantly, does not want to come back for a recurrence.

HISTOPATHOLOGY PITFALLS

Though BCC is usually readily identifiable with intraoperative frozen sections, there are some cases in which difficulties arise and these are a significant cause of error.

General difficulties may include histologic interpretation of highly infiltrative BCC, BCC with extensive perineural invasion, and BCC obfuscated by dense infiltrates of leukemia or chronic inflammation. In such cases, an additional safety margin may be taken following complete excision to allow confirmation of this margin with paraffin section examination. Immunohistochemistry with p63 or a cytokeratin can also be used to highlight subtle carcinoma. Alternatively, if the difficulties are obvious preoperatively, the entire margin assessment can be performed with formalin-fixed paraffin processing (slow Mohs). Given that this generally takes a minimum of 24 hours to process, the surgeon needs to decide whether to close/reconstruct directly or dress the open wound until the margins are confirmed to be negative.

In addition to these general difficulties, there are several entities which may mimic BCC, leading to misdiagnosis in the preoperative biopsy or misinterpretation intraoperatively. Due to the consequent risk of unnecessary further excisions, these are worth emphasizing (**Figs. 8.14 to 8.24**).

"Folliculocentric basaloid proliferation" is an umbrella term that attempts to define a range of abnormal follicular proliferations which are sometimes misdiagnosed as BCC. This was first described in a group of patients undergoing Mohs micrographic surgery (MMS) for nasal and perinasal BCC; however, the frequency is unreported. There is a wide range of patterns, and some of the reported cases likely represent incidental benign follicular tumors (e.g., pilar sheath acanthoma). Histology shows a uniform basal cell proliferation with surrounding normal stroma.[7]

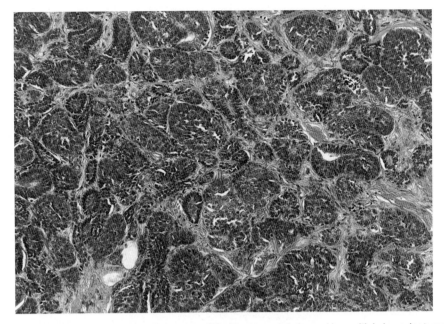

FIGURE 8.14. Cylindroma shows a nonencapsulated tumor nodule formed by multiple irregular tumor islands, arranged in an aptly named "jigsaw" pattern. Surrounding the tumor islands is a thick hyaline deposition. Two populations of cells are noted to make up the tumor nodules: A smaller cell with a hyperchromatic nucleus tending to the periphery, and larger cells with open nuclei throughout the center of the nodules. These features and the lack of retraction artifact help distinguish this tumor from BCC.

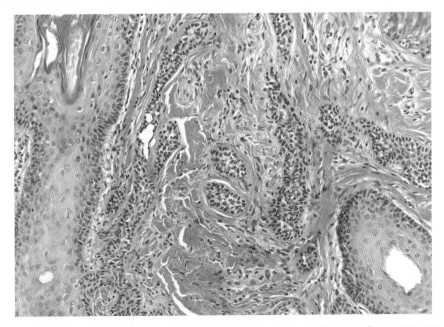

FIGURE 8.15. Proliferations of the mantle area of the sebaceous apparatus are quite common on facial skin and may mimic BCC. These form thin strands of basaloid cells emanating from the base of the infundibulum of hairs. They can be identified by the pattern and the identification of intermixed sebaceous cells seen at higher magnification.

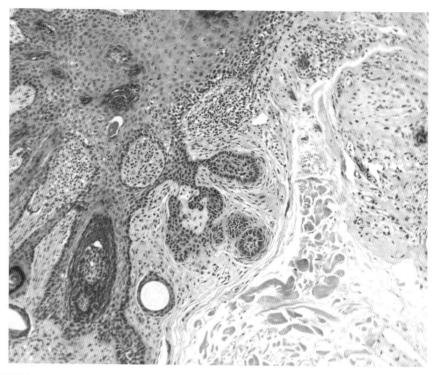

FIGURE 8.16. In trichofolliculoma, numerous small follicles radiate from a central larger follicle. The hairs are surrounded by a well-circumscribed dense stroma. The surrounding hairs are generally very small (vellus).

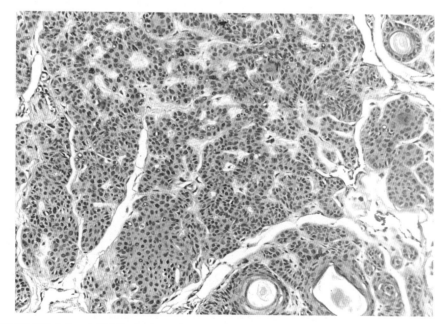

FIGURE 8.17. In basaloid follicular hamartoma, there are anastomosing strands of basaloid and squamoid cells with connection to the overlying epithelium. The cells are bland, without atypia, and show a loose, cellular, or myxoid stroma. Retraction artifact is generally not seen.

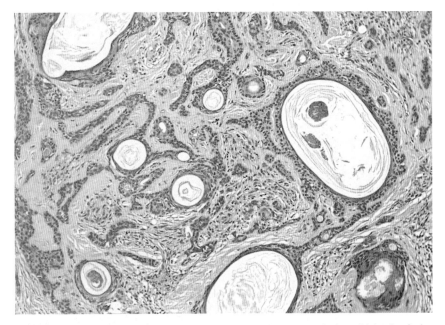

FIGURE 8.18. **In desmoplastic trichoepithelioma, the tumor is composed of small islands of a basaloid tumor superficially which form cords and strands toward the base and periphery.** Horn cysts, calcification, and foreign-body granulomas can be seen. The cells are bland and mitotic activity is usually very low; however, the infiltrative sclerosing growth pattern can cause difficulty in discriminating this lesion from carcinoma.

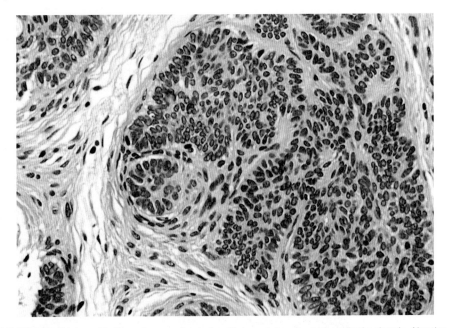

FIGURE 8.19. **Trichoepithelioma is comprised of multiple nodules situated within the dermis.** Abortive hair follicles and calcifications are frequently seen. The stroma is denser and more cellular than with BCC, and there is often focal stromal cracking as opposed to retraction artifact seen in BCC. Trichoblastoma is composed of larger nests than trichoepithelioma. The lack of prominent cleft retraction, lack of significant mitotic activity, and absence of cytologic atypia help distinguish these benign follicular tumors from BCC.

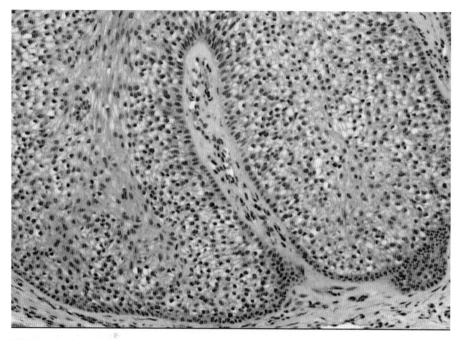

FIGURE 8.20. The key finding in trichilemmoma is a downgrowth of epithelial cells with increasing clear cell differentiation and basal peripheral palisading surrounded by eosinophilic hyaline basement membrane.

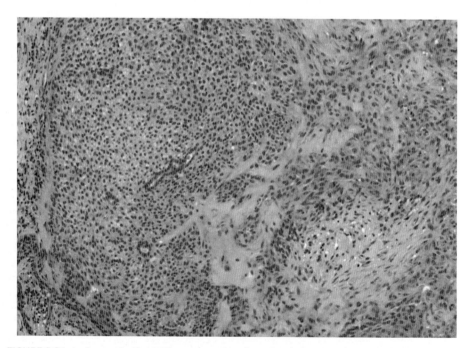

FIGURE 8.21. In desmoplastic trichilemmoma, the tumor develops infiltrating cords predominantly at the base of the lesion. Key to the diagnosis is recognition of a sclerotic dermis/basement membrane between the tumor cords. Clear cells as seen in regular trichilemmoma are a constant feature.

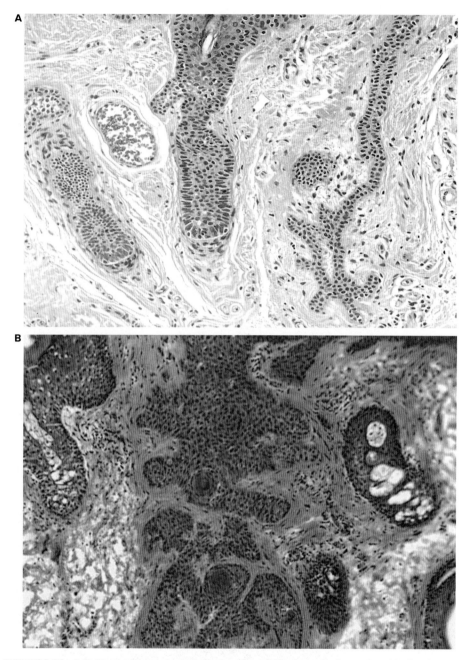

FIGURE 8.22. A, B: The facial area has a high density of follicular and sebaceous epithelia which can look unusual in some sections. Following these areas through multiple microscopic sections can help to conclude that these are unusual follicles rather than foci of carcinoma.

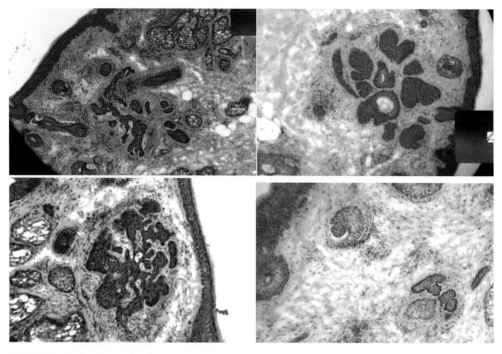

FIGURE 8.23. Four examples of follicular basaloid proliferation which may mimic BCC. There is a uniform basal cell proliferation surrounded by a normal stroma. There is no retraction. The image on the top right may be an incidental pilar sheath acanthoma. Some authors recommend reviewing multiple levels to better define the proliferation and to take an additional level of the area if it is present at the margin.

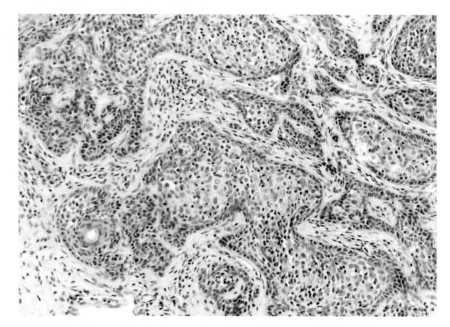

FIGURE 8.24. In cutaneous lymphadenoma, there is a well-circumscribed dermal mass composed of basaloid tumor islands infiltrated by populations of lymphocytes. As with other benign tumors, the surrounding stroma is fibrotic and intimately connected to the epithelial islands.

SUMMARY

BCC is an ideal tumor for MCS with excellent cure rates. Having a system which stratifies risk helps in surgical planning. This system should consider the histopathology revealed by the biopsy as well as patient factors. The main challenge in dealing with these common tumors is histologically mistaking BCC for other tumors or benign native structures.

References

1. Smeets NWJ, Krekels GAM, Ostertag JU, et al. Surgical excision vs Mohs' micrographic surgery for basal-cell carcinoma of the face: randomised controlled trial. *Lancet*. 2004;364:1766-1772.
2. Mosterd K, Krekels GAM, Nieman FH, et al. Surgical excision versus Mohs' micrographic surgery for primary and recurrent basal-cell carcinoma of the face: a prospective randomised controlled trial with 5-years follow-up. *Lancet Oncol*. 2008;9:1149-1156.
3. Boehringer A, Adam P, Schnabl S, et al. Analysis of incomplete excisions of basal-cell carcinomas after breadloaf microscopy compared with 3D-microscopy: a prospective randomized and blinded study. *J Cutan Pathol*. 2015;42:542-553.
4. van Loo E, Mosterd K, Krekels GA, et al. Surgical excision versus Mohs' micrographic surgery for basal cell carcinoma of the face: a randomised clinical trial with 10-year follow-up. *Eur J Cancer*. 2014;50(17):3011-3020.
5. McKenzie CA, Chen AC, Choy B, Fernández-Peñas P, Damian DL, Scolyer RA. Classification of high risk basal cell carcinoma subtypes: experience of the ONTRAC study with proposed definitions and guidelines for pathological reporting. *Pathology*. 2016;48(5):395-397.
6. Nedved D, Tonkovic-Capin V, Hunt E, et al. Diagnostic concordance rates in the subtyping of basal cell carcinoma by different dermatopathologists. *J Cutan Pathol*. 2014;41(1):9-13.
7. Anjum N, Robson A, Craythorne E, Mallipeddi R. Follicular proliferation or basal cell carcinoma? The first prospective U.K. study of this histological challenge during Mohs surgery. *Br J Dermatol*. 2017;177(2):549-550.

9

Cutaneous Squamous Cell Carcinoma

Patrick Emanuel / Garrett Desman

Burden
Evidence
Clinical Presentation
Biopsy
Risk Stratification and Histopathology
    Perineural Invasion
Debulk

Multidisciplinary Consultation
Pitfalls
    Concurrent Lymphoproliferative Disease
    Metastasis Versus Primary SCC
    Sialometaplasia or Syringometaplasia
Safety Margins
Summary

BURDEN

An argument could be made that cutaneous squamous cell carcinoma (cSCC) is a neglected cancer globally. cSCC imposes a significant disease burden on health care systems, with an estimated 250,000 cases diagnosed annually in the United States. Yet, its true incidence is difficult to decipher as it is not generally recorded in tumor registries. Some statistics are frankly alarming.[1]

The burden has shown a dramatic increase over recent decades. Metastases and deaths from cSCC are still regarded by many as *black swan* events. Black swan events represent extreme outliers (outside the sphere of normal to such a degree that nothing in the past suggests its possibility), result in an acute impact, and are only explainable following the event. But cSCC disease burden is increasing both in terms of incidence *and* mortality to such an extent that deaths from cSCC have been estimated to exceed those caused by melanoma in some populations. The increase has been attributed largely to cumulative sun exposure, the advent of new immunosuppression therapies, and organ transplantation.

Like the underappreciation of disease burden, research interest in and funding for cSCC lags behind that of other malignancies. The lack of available tumor material is a significant barrier to research. A typical patient with metastatic cSCC has innumerable possible primary tumors and deciphering which one was responsible for the metastasis can be impossible. This is not frequently discussed and, disappointingly, many studies looking into risk use pathology reports without slide review or proper consideration of which skin tumor is responsible for the metastatic disease.[2]

Margin control surgery (MCS) is an attractive therapeutic option. cSCC has a propensity to occur on cosmetically and functionally sensitive sun-damaged skin; it usually grows in a predictable cohesive pattern; usually has a recognizable histopathology; and complete excision is usually associated with an excellent prognosis.

EVIDENCE

To date, no comprehensive randomized control trials or prospective cohort studies have been performed which compare MCS with other treatment modalities. In a systematic review of the literature since 1940, Rowe et al. reported a five-year local recurrence rate of 3.1% ($n = 2065$) for primary cSCC treated with MCS and a rate of 8.1% for WLE. When high-risk factors were considered, MCS has shown even more favorable outcomes: a local recurrence rate of 25.2% versus 41.7% for tumors 2 cm or larger, 32.6% versus 53.6% for poorly differentiated cSCC, and 0% versus 47% for neurotropic cSCC. For recurrent cSCC, the meta-analysis by Rowe et al. revealed a five-year recurrence rate after MCS of 10.0% ($n = 151$) compared with 23.3% ($n = 34$) following WLE.[3-6]

CLINICAL PRESENTATION

cSCC has quite a wide range of clinical presentations. Thin lesions are often erythematous scaly papules or plaques. Thicker tumors typically present as an indurated erythematous plaque, nodule, or ulcer. Invasive tumors are often surrounded by actinic keratosis (AK) (**Fig. 9.1**).

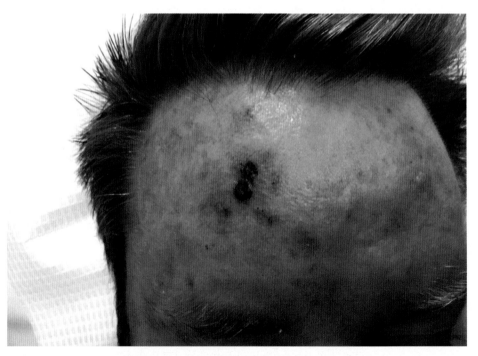

FIGURE 9.1. Centrally, there is invasive cSCC which is indurated and has focal ulceration. Around this is a broad area of erythema and scale consistent with AK. Given its indistinct radial borders and occurrence on cosmetically sensitive skin, this is an ideal carcinoma for MCS.

BIOPSY

All cases need to be biopsied to confirm the clinical diagnosis. Generally (independent of patient factors), thinner nonindurated tumors can be sampled by shave biopsy. If deep invasion is suspected, a punch biopsy or a deep incisional biopsy may be more appropriate. Scouting biopsies to get a handle on the size of the process may be helpful for some poorly defined lesions, or for recurrent tumors within scars from previous reconstructions.

The histopathology biopsy report needs to be more comprehensive than simply diagnosing the tumor as cSCC. Historically, extremely brief diagnostic reports were the norm and these often did not mention key features such as depth of invasion or aggressive morphology. Encouraging discussion between the pathologist and the surgeon may help to change this practice. The pathologist should report histopathologic risk factors which include the data points necessary for the staging system chosen in their community. Typically, these include depth of invasion, thickness of the tumor (mm), differentiation, invasion of nerves, and mention of an unusual morphology. It may help the pathologist to know that slightly more comprehensive reports may aid in decision-making. The additional time and effort required for the pathologist to change their practice are minimal.

Clinical features raising the concern of perineural infiltration need to be taken seriously. These include tingling, numbness, pain, or loss of motor control. In these cases, a larger (often deeper) biopsy to prove perineural invasion is useful prior to excision (**Figs. 9.2** and **9.3**). High-resolution MRI can help assess significant nerve invasion.

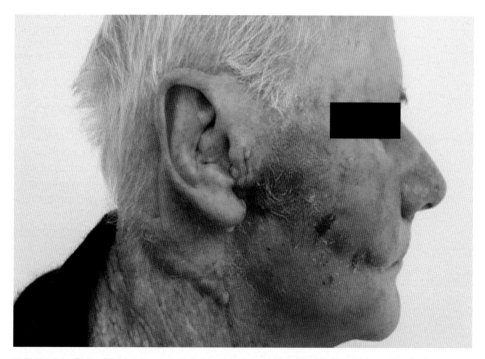

FIGURE 9.2. **This cSCC had recurred at the site of previous wide local excision and radiotherapy.** Recurrence included facial nerve involvement. An MRI scan confirmed that the patient had a noted facial nerve deficit and neurotropic disease extensively involving the facial nerve. Multiple incisional skin biopsies confirmed dermal and subcutaneous deposits of SCC-invading nerves.

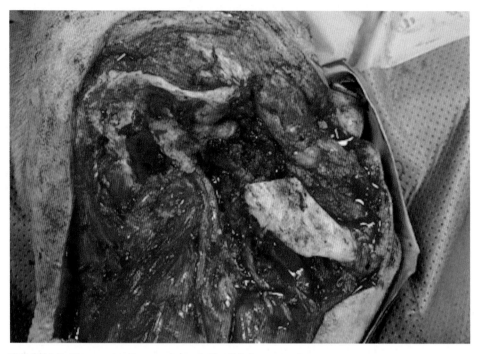

FIGURE 9.3. **The same patient as shown in Fig. 9.2**. Intraoperative margins were examined *en face* with frozen sections. The tumor extended along the facial nerve branches and approached the lateral canthus but did not involve the orbit, which could be spared. Large, complicated cSCCs can benefit from a complete intraoperative margin assessment which guides the size and shape of the required excision. The confidence given by performing a complete excision intraoperatively before embarking on a complex reconstruction can be invaluable.

RISK STRATIFICATION AND HISTOPATHOLOGY

Risk is usually stratified using current protocols (e.g., AJCC, NCCN, BWH; see Chap. 4). Clinical metrics usually considered important for risk are summarized in **Table 9.1**.

cSCC is composed histologically of malignant keratinocytes which infiltrate the dermis. An associated precursor lesion (AK or SCC in situ) is often present.

cSCC is generally graded in a three-tier system: Well-, moderately, or poorly differentiated depending on the degree of keratinization (**Figs. 9.4** to **9.7**). Anaplastic, undifferentiated, or sarcomatoid tumors may be lumped together with poorly differentiated tumors. There is considerable subjectivity in this system which is probably why it is not mentioned

---

TABLE 9.1 Main Clinical Risk Factors

- Tumor size
- Immunosuppression (HIV, hematologic malignancy, pharmacologic immunosuppression, and organ transplant recipients)
- High-risk anatomic site
- Recurrent tumors
- Radiotherapy
- Genetic syndrome (e.g., xeroderma pigmentosum)

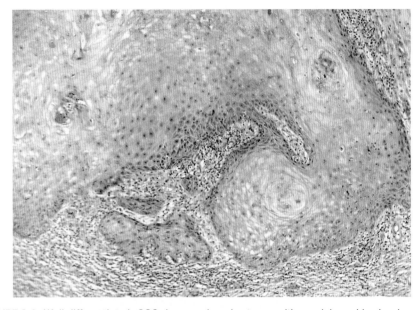

FIGURE 9.4. **Well-differentiated cSCC shows an invasive tumor with a mainly pushing border and prominent keratinization.** The tumor cells undergo maturation so that the tumor mimics the epithelium of normal epidermis. There is minimal cytologic atypia.

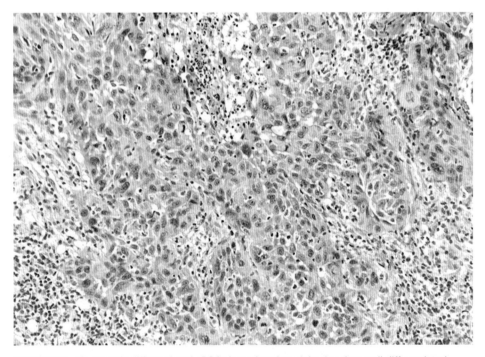

FIGURE 9.5. **Moderately differentiated cSCC shows less keratinization than well-differentiated tumors but the keratinization is quite easy to find.** These tumors usually have a more infiltrative growth pattern. Careful examination for invasion of nerves or vessels is warranted.

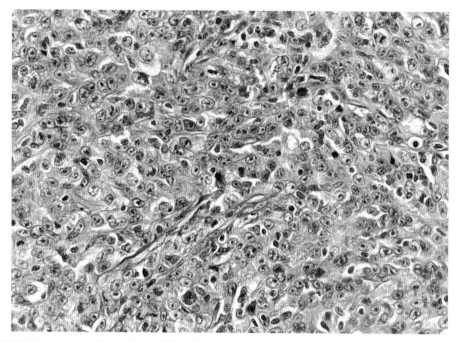

FIGURE 9.6. **Poorly differentiated cSCC is considered high-risk in the NCCN.** These tumors show little evidence of squamous differentiation of routine sections. IHC is often needed to prove squamous differentiation.

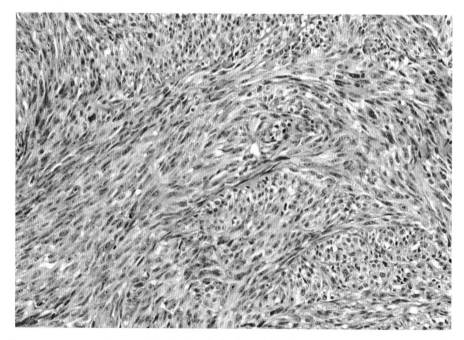

FIGURE 9.7. **cSCC with sarcomatoid differentiation is considered a high-risk phenotype by the NCCN.** This example shows large malignant spindled cells with no evidence of keratinization. IHC is needed to exclude melanoma or sarcoma.

TABLE 9.2 Main Histology Risk Factors

- Risk morphology (e.g., poorly differentiated, sarcomatoid, desmoplastic)
- Perineural invasion
- Deep invasion

---

in some of the staging protocols. Some authors have advocated a two-tier system (well- to moderately differentiated or poorly differentiated), similar to the systems adopted in other organ systems (e.g., urothelial). There are numerous other histologic risk metrics which may be seen in the various staging protocols and appropriate use documents. The main metrics are summarized in **Table 9.2**.

In addition to the grading system, there is a variety of recognized morphologic cSCC variants which carry a greater risk. These variants represent dedifferentiation or trans-differentiation of the keratinocytes of cSCC which, mechanistically, is probably akin to what occurs in poorly differentiated or anaplastic tumors. The most recognized variants include adenosquamous, desmoplastic, acantholytic, clear cell, and lymphoepithelial carcinoma (**Figs. 9.8** to **9.10**). Some of these morphologies may only come to light during MCS. Unfortunately, the definitions of these variants are subject to subjectivity and the literature is not comprehensive in proving that some are associated with a higher risk.

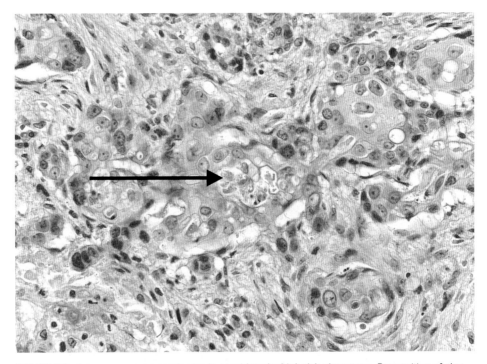

FIGURE 9.8. Adenosquamous carcinoma is considered a high-risk phenotype. Recognition of glandular differentiation (arrow) within a cSCC points to this diagnosis.

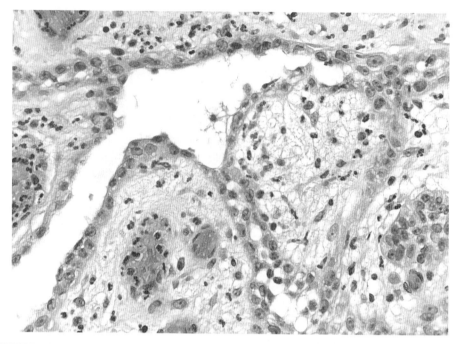

FIGURE 9.9. **Acantholytic cSCC is composed of keratinocytes which lack cell-to-cell connections between keratinocytes, so the tumor appears to fall apart.** Sometimes this imparts a morphology which can mimic glandular differentiation.

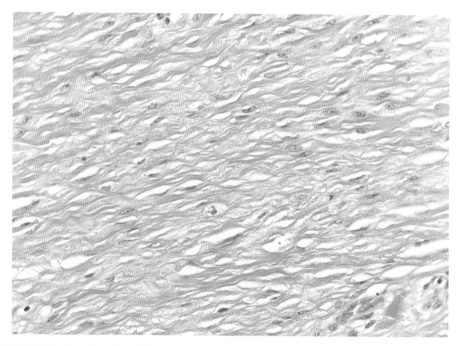

FIGURE 9.10. **Desmoplastic cSCC shows subtle infiltrating carcinoma cells invading a sclerotic/desmoplastic stroma.** These tumors can be subtle histologically and resemble a hypertrophic scar.

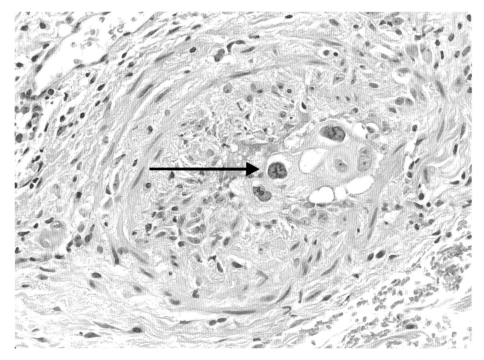

FIGURE 9.11. Lymphatic or vascular (arrow) invasion of cSCC is not commonly seen and likely frequently overlooked.

Invasion of lymphovascular spaces implies a significantly greater risk. Though this metric shows one of the most striking correlations with increased risk of recurrence, metastasis, and death of disease, it is in fact rarely seen, which may be why it is not included in most of the staging protocols[7] (**Fig. 9.11**).

Perineural Invasion

Perineural invasion (PNI) implies risk. In the most recent AJCC (8th edition), the involved nerves were further defined as either being greater than 0.1 mm in diameter or within the subcutaneous tissue (**Fig. 9.12**).

Though PNI usually spreads along the perineural space in a contiguous fashion, sometimes a connection between the main tumor and a large nerve may not seem contiguous (**Fig. 9.13**). This has led to the suggestion that some cases of perineural invasion represent metastasis. Perineural metastasis at least partly explains why cases with PNI seem to benefit from adjuvant radiotherapy, even following what is thought to be a complete surgical excision.

It was historically believed that PNI represented lymphatic spread of tumor into nerves or that the nerve sheath represents a low-resistance path for tumor spread. But definitive studies have proven an absence of lymphatics within the inner sanctum of the nerve sheath, and several layers of collagen and basement membrane wrap around the inside of the nerve, so this is not a low-resistance path. Evidence is emerging that indicates that PNI is more like invasion than simple diffusion, with models showing signaling between the nerves and invading tumor cells.[8]

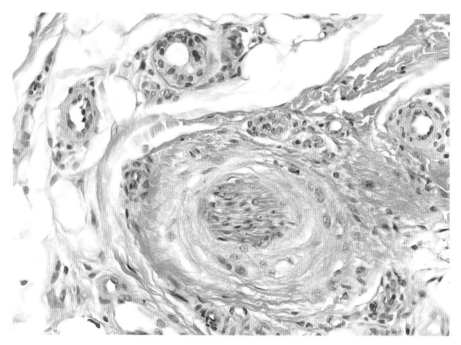

FIGURE 9.12. Perineural infiltration involving nerves in the subcutis or nerves larger than 0.1 mm are considered very high risk by NCCN.

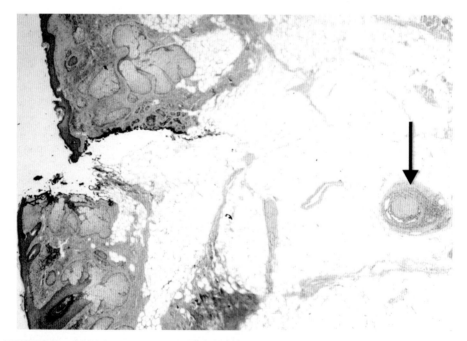

FIGURE 9.13. cSCC in a subcutaneous nerve discontinuous from the main tumor mass. The zone between the main tumor and this nerve was entirely examined *en face* and proved there is no connection between this focus and the main tumor.

DEBULK

Before performing the excision of the first level, the tumor is frequently debulked. Instead of a curettage debulk, it is often advisable to excise the central debulk specimen with a scalpel and send this for paraffin section examination. This paraffin specimen helps assess thickness, pattern, morphology, and the presence of perineural or lymphovascular invasion. Such an assessment is particularly necessary for cases in which the biopsy does not appear to be representative of the entire tumor.

Molecular testing may also be performed on this debulk specimen if needed. These tests may serve as prognostic markers or for therapeutic options. For example, Castle Bioscience's DecisionDx® is a gene expression assay (qRT-PCR) that stratifies risk into categories and can only be performed on paraffin-embedded tissue. The debulk specimen can also serve for research purposes.

MULTIDISCIPLINARY CONSULTATION

Multidisciplinary consultation and management are recommended for patients with a high risk of locoregional or distant metastases. Deciding which patients may benefit from these is a challenge. Whichever triage system is chosen, applying a protocol within a community is helpful in achieving consistency of care.

PITFALLS

Though most cases are straightforward, an incomplete excision or underestimating the significance of nerve invasion can lead to significant problems. It is true that fewer histopathologic mimics exist for cSCC than with basal cell carcinoma (BCC), but sometimes the histopathology is far from clear. Subtle fronts of invasive tumor may be challenging to say the least, with some cases being extremely difficult to interpret without the aid of IHC.

Overlooking subtle infiltrating areas of carcinoma may have devastating consequences. In Dostoevsky's masterpiece *Crime and Punishment,* the protagonist Raskolnikov's internal struggle is much like the struggle faced by a pathologist who makes a significant diagnostic error. Raskolnikov commits murder with the idea that he possesses enough intellectual and emotional fortitude to deal with the ramifications. The pathologist who has significant experience and skill scans a slide quickly and overlooks a minute focus of cSCC in a nerve in the subcutis, far away from the main tumor mass. Raskolnikov's sense of guilt soon overwhelms him to the point of psychological and physical illness. The pathologist discovers the patient has returned months later with disease in the nerves of the skull base and sleepless nights ensue. Raskolnikov confesses and accepts his formal punishment. The pathologist reviews the previous slides, sees that they missed the carcinoma, and knows that they too must admit culpability (**Fig. 9.14**).

Some of the aggressive histopathologic growth patterns may be poorly visualized with frozen sections (e.g., sarcomatoid/spindle cell or single-cell infiltrative cSCC), which may limit the utility of MCS. It is important to be aware of these difficulties at the time of MCS by reviewing the biopsy slides preoperatively (**Fig. 9.15**).

Concurrent Lymphoproliferative Disease

Admixed lymphoma within cSCC can cause difficulties in the interpretation of the histopathologic slides. Firstly, the lymphomatous infiltrates can be mistaken for reactive (benign) inflammatory infiltrates. The most encountered lymphoproliferative disease

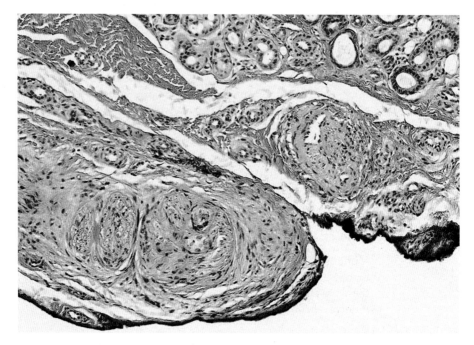

FIGURE 9.14. **cSCC invading a nerve.** Missing these foci during margin assessment can have disastrous consequences.

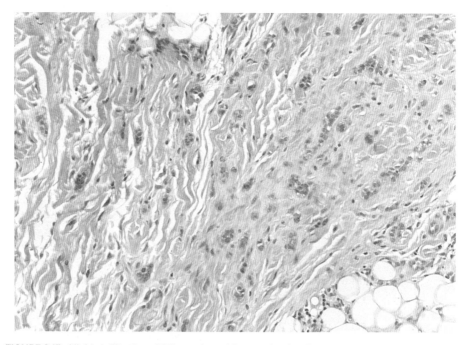

FIGURE 9.15. **Highly infiltrative cSCC can show thin strands of malignant cells or even single tumor cells invading deeply.** Such cases may benefit from a final safety margin or intraoperative IHC margin assessment.

is chronic lymphocytic leukemia. Key to the recognition of this is the identification of dense lymphocytic infiltrates intermixed with the cSCC. The lymphocytes are small and monotonous without the variable size and shape typical of a benign lymphocytic infiltrate. Almost invariably, benign infiltrates in the skin are predominantly composed of T cells. Dense infiltrates of B cells should alert the pathologist to a possible B cell lymphoma and warrant a wider panel of immunohistochemical markers. Secondly, patients with known lymphoma have the propensity to develop high-risk cSCC, so many of these cases will show a high-risk morphology which may also be challenging (subtle and highly infiltrative) histopathologically. The carcinoma may be obfuscated to the point of being almost impossible to see without IHC (**Figs. 9.16** and **9.17**). In such cases, a paraffin safety margin may be helpful in adding another layer of confidence following a clearance of the tumor with frozen section examination.

Metastasis Versus Primary SCC

Occasionally, it can be difficult to know whether a tumor is a primary cSCC or metastasis from a secondary cSCC from another site. This is particularly the case in high-risk patients with a previous history of multiple carcinomas and other risk factors (e.g., immunosuppression). While the presence of intraepidermal involvement can be helpful in identifying a carcinoma as a primary tumor, ulceration and direct invasion of the overlying epidermis can cause confusion. A history of previous metastasis and location in the vicinity of a previous high-risk carcinoma should raise suspicions. Sometimes, the suspicion only arises during MCS when the pattern of invasion suggests a tumor based in the deeper tissues such as the parotid.

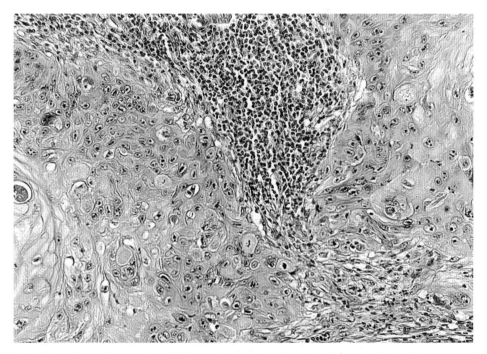

FIGURE 9.16. **cSCC with intermixed chronic lymphocytic leukemia is seen in the upper aspect of this photo.** Lymphomas may occasionally be first diagnosed in a biopsy specimen of cSCC or during MCS.

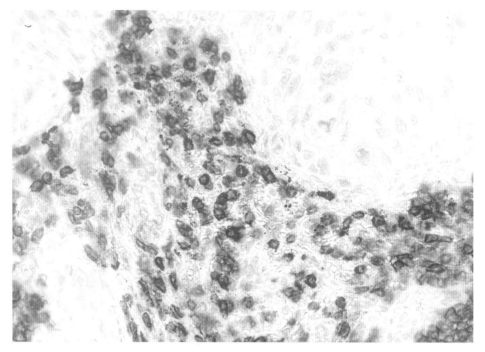

FIGURE 9.17. IHC with CD20 shows dense infiltrates of positive cells consistent with a B cell population. In contrast, benign lymphoid infiltrates are predominantly composed of CD20-negative T cells.

Sialometaplasia or Syringometaplasia

Regenerative changes in salivary glands (sialometaplasia) or sweat glands (syringometaplasia) may cause squamous metaplasia which can mimic cSCC. There may be profound nuclear atypia, especially in patients with a history of previous radiotherapy. Clues to distinguish this benign reaction from cSCC include recognition that the architecture is lobular and that the squamous cells are colonizing a benign gland (**Fig. 9.18**).

SAFETY MARGINS

A final rim of margin taken following intraoperative margin clearance helps in cases where the cSCC is difficult to see in frozen sections (**Figs. 9.19** and **9.20**). This is particularly helpful for cases with subtle perineural invasion. IHC with p63, p40, or cytokeratin (usually CK5/6) can serve as an adjunct to highlight subtle carcinoma.

SUMMARY

While MCS is generally an excellent treatment option for cSCC, the surgeon needs to be cognizant that some cases display an aggressive behavior. Consideration of the biopsy technique and the need for a debulk specimen help to stage tumors accurately. cSCC has quite a diversity of morphologies and assessment of surgical margins can be a challenge. Critically, meticulous attention is needed to exclude PNI and minimize the chance of a poor outcome.

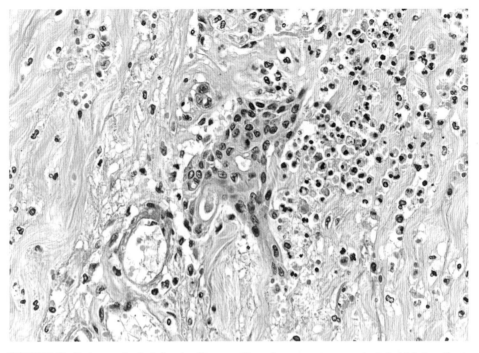

FIGURE 9.18. **Syringometaplasia in a healing scar.** There is some squamous atypia but this is uniform and the clue to distinguish this benign reaction from cSCC is recognition of a residual normal eccrine duct.

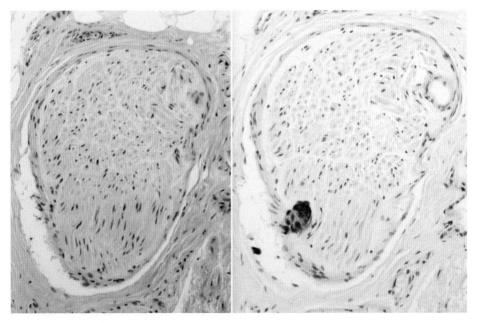

FIGURE 9.19. **Cytokeratin IHC can be a useful adjunct in the assessment of the margins to exclude subtle residual disease.** In this example, there is no carcinoma in the HE section of the peripheral nerve but subsequent immunohistochemical examination for cytokeratin revealed neural invasion (right).

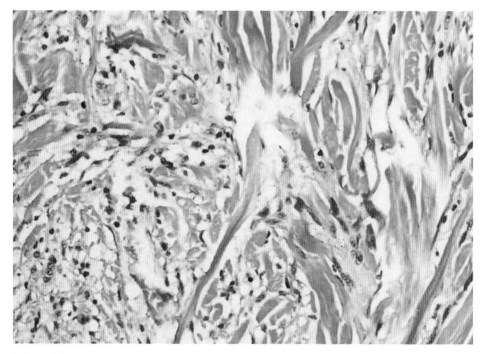

FIGURE 9.20. A safety margin can be helpful in subtle carcinomas such as this desmoplastic cSCC. These are difficult to distinguish from scars when performing frozen section examination.

References

1. Pondicherry A, Martin R, Meredith I, Rolfe J, Emanuel P, Elwood M. The burden of non-melanoma skin cancers in Auckland, New Zealand. *Australas J Dermatol.* 2018;59(3):210-213.
2. Agar NJ, Kirton C, Patel RS, Martin RC, Angelo N, Emanuel PO. Predicting lymph node metastases in cutaneous squamous cell carcinoma: use of a morphological scoring system. *N Z Med J.* 2015;128(1411):59-67.
3. Lawrence N, Cottel WI. Squamous cell carcinoma of skin with perineural invasion. *J Am Acad Dermatol.* 1994;31(1):30-33.
4. Leibovitch I, Huilgol SC, Selva D, Hill D, Richards S, Paver R. Cutaneous squamous cell carcinoma treated with Mohs micrographic surgery in Australia I. Experience over 10 years. *J Am Acad Dermatol.* 2005;53(2):253-260.
5. Rowe DE, Carroll RJ, Day CL Jr. Prognostic factors for local recurrence, metastasis, and survival rates in squamous cell carcinoma of the skin, ear, and lip. Implications for treatment modality selection. *J Am Acad Dermatol.* 1992;26(6):976-990.
6. Stuart SE, Schoen P, Jin C, et al. Tumor recurrence of keratinocyte carcinomas judged appropriate for Mohs micrographic surgery using appropriate use criteria. *J Am Acad Dermatol.* 2017;76(6):1131-1138.
7. Thompson AK, Kelley BF, Prokop LJ, Murad MH, Baum CL. Risk factors for cutaneous squamous cell carcinoma recurrence, metastasis, and disease-specific death: a systematic review and meta-analysis. *JAMA Dermatol.* 2016;152(4):419-428.
8. Liebig C, Ayala G, Wilks JA, Berger DH, Albo D. Perineural invasion in cancer: a review of the literature. *Cancer.* 2009;115(15):3379-3391.

10

Melanoma

Patrick Emanuel / Gonzalo Ziegler-Rodriguez

Suitability
Efficacy
Biopsy
Debulk
Control Biopsy
The First Level
Specimen Processing Techniques

MMS
Modified MMS
Hybrid Technique
Management of Massive Invasive Melanoma
"Mapped" Excision
Histopathology
Summary

One of the hallmarks of the natural world is variation. For instance, the spectrum of visible light is infinitely varied, and though the difference between the blinding sunlight of midday and the impenetrable blackness of an underground cave is stark, between these extremes lie gradations that the eye cannot always distinguish. Similarly, a key issue faced when assessing the margins of lentigo maligna (LM) is to determine whether melanocytes represent the periphery of melanoma *or* background melanocytes on sun-damaged skin.

Despite strong resistance in some surgical circles, the use of margin control surgery (MCS) for treating melanoma is increasing. A range of methods has been described in the literature and this has muddied the waters somewhat, which may explain some of this resistance.

SUITABILITY

Though MCS has been used for thick invasive melanoma, the NCCN and various working groups continue to recommend a traditional wide local excision (WLE) in accordance with the established margin guidelines rather than MCS for these invasive cases. Until further studies are published, it seems prudent to generally abide by these guidelines in which the size of the excision margin is determined by the thickness of the invasive melanoma.

MCS for melanoma in situ (MIS) has gained popularity and wider acceptance in the community. Almost all the literature refers to the treatment of head and neck MIS of the LM type, but MCS has also been used quite widely for other forms of MIS (particularly for cases where excision is difficult in accordance with the recommended margin size). MCS for *minimally invasive* melanoma on anatomically constrained sites (e.g., the face, nose, acral sites) is currently included in the NCCN. The use of MCS in this context is recommended to include a comprehensive histologic assessment, which is usually a final paraffin margin assessment with dermatopathology review.[1,2]

LM is a form of MIS which commonly occurs on sun-exposed skin of the head and neck in the elderly. It represents the precursor lesion of invasive lentigo maligna melanoma (LMM). Like all forms of melanoma, the rate of progressing from in situ disease (LM) to invasive disease (LMM) is unknown. Given that some cases of LM may persist without invasion for a very long time, historically it was not considered a form of MIS. More recent acceptance that LM will evolve into invasive LMM if the patient lives long enough has changed this sentiment, and characterization of LM as a form of MIS has become almost universally accepted. Destructive and chemical therapies may be useful in selected patients and lesions, but surgical excision with meticulous histologic examination of the margins produces the highest cure rate.

The currently recommended surgical margins for MIS generally range from 0.5 to 1 cm. Unfortunately, these margin recommendations are often not sufficient for LM on the head and neck. With the goal of achieving negative margins 97% of the time, surgical margins of up to 12 mm for in situ lesions on the head/neck have been recommended.[3] This is a key reason for choosing MCS; usually the tumor is microscopically much smaller than this, yet sometimes it extends further than 12 mm from the clinically visible tumor. Avoiding this *guesswork* is the central goal of MCS. Factors driving the popularity of MCS for LM are summarized in **Table 10.1**.

EFFICACY

There is significant evidence that MCS is effective for MIS. A recent review reported recurrence rates of 1.35% with MCS, which compares with 5% to 20% in LM excised by WLE. Another review comparing Mohs micrographic surgery (MMS) with WLE showed 1.9% and 5.9% recurrence rates, respectively. The recurrence rate of the hybrid (frozen section and paraffin) technique is comparable (1%).[4] Johnson's square MCS method revealed a 0.9% recurrence rate, all occurring within the first year.[2] A recent retrospective analysis of 277 patients treated with MMS and 385 patients treated with conventional wide excision (WE) (mean surgical margins, 0.6 cm) demonstrated no significant differences in local recurrence rates, overall survival, or melanoma-specific survival at a median follow-up of 8.6 years. Other retrospective analyses and prospectively followed cohorts have demonstrated lower rates of local recurrence for LM on the face and ears with MCS.[2]

BIOPSY

It is generally recommended that the initial biopsy of melanoma should be an excisional biopsy, which may be a punch excision, shave excision, or elliptical excision. For larger facial lesions, however, this may not be feasible. For large flat pigmented lesions, a biopsy

---

TABLE 10.1 Factors Driving MCS for MIS

- LM is characterized by an unpredictable, subclinical extension beyond the visible pigmented and Wood's lamp margins (**Fig. 10.1**)
- Recommended surgical margins (up to 12 mm for LM on the head and neck) which may not be feasible on cosmetically sensitive skin
- The frustration felt by the patient and surgeon alike when faced with positive margins for a tumor which has been excised and closed or reconstructed
- The significant number of early and late (5-10 years) local recurrences after WLE surgery for LM
- Ease of the technique given the expertise gained in treating other cutaneous tumors with MCS

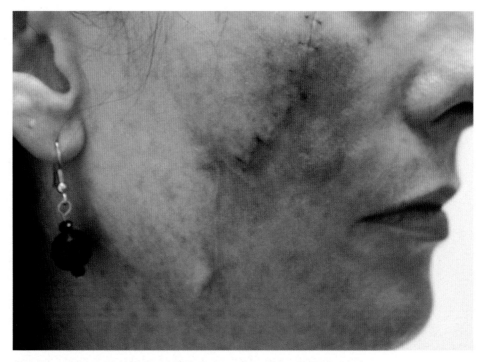

FIGURE 10.1. This large amelanotic MIS illustrates the utility of MCS for melanoma. This patient had two previous excisions with standard bread loaf sections with positive margins. The outline of the tumor was impossible to discern with Wood's lamp and dermoscopy. MCS guided the extent of the excision needed for complete removal.

that permits maximum histopathologic examination of the epidermis is needed. This is usually a broad shave biopsy (which in many cases actually serves as an excisional biopsy). Broad shave biopsies have the additional benefit of providing an excellent cosmetic result in the case that the lesion is benign (e.g., macular seborrheic keratosis, lentigo simplex). If invasion is suspected, a deeper incisional biopsy is needed. For large lesions, the most clinically atypical area should be biopsied, but if the lesion is completely uniform, it is helpful to have the biopsy include some normal epidermis in the periphery so that comparison between lesional and nonlesional skin can be appreciated histologically. Small, partial punch biopsies have a very limited role and are a frequent cause for misdiagnosis (the authors have seen more melanomas misdiagnosed with punch biopsies of flat facial lesions than in any other context; **Fig. 10.2**).

DEBULK

Key to the success of MCS for melanoma is debulking of the tumor with a scalpel (not curettage) for examination in regular vertical paraffin sections. This is critically important for diagnostic and staging purposes. The reasons for this are summarized in **Table 10.2**.

There are three options: The surgeon removes the debulk prior to removing the margin, *or* the debulk is removed from the specimen following excision, *or* the tumor is removed following clearance of the peripheral strips of radial margin.

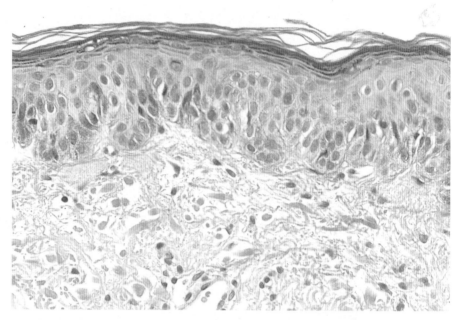

FIGURE 10.2. **Some areas of LM have very little evidence of melanocytic proliferation.** This area has all the features of solar lentigo with basal hypermelanosis and elongation of rete ridges. If small punch biopsies are performed on LM, there is always a risk that areas without much melanocytic proliferation are sampled, leading erroneously to a benign diagnosis.

TABLE 10.2 Reasons for a Debulk of MIS Specimens

- It is not uncommon for a biopsy to have been diagnosed as MIS, only to have invasion discovered at the time of complete excision. Various studies have reported invasive malignancy found in the debulk in 5%-18% of cases of excisions for LM.
- The thickness of the invasive melanoma is impossible to measure if it is not processed routinely in vertical sections. Other metrics such as satellitosis, lymphovascular invasion, and mitotic rate may be impossible to assess without standard vertical sections.
- Invasive melanoma can be extremely subtle. For example, desmoplastic melanoma frequently occurs in the dermis underneath LM and may resemble a scar or other benign lesion histologically (**Figs. 10.3** and **10.4**).

CONTROL BIOPSY

Some teams favor processing a specimen of contralateral skin to act as a baseline for the density of melanocytes. Others find this unnecessary, as background melanocytic populations can be readily assessed during microscopic assessment of the entire radial margin which should consist of predominantly normal background skin.

THE FIRST LEVEL

A wider first level is generally excised for melanoma than for nonmelanoma skin cancer. A nonstandard 6-mm margin around the clinically visible tumor is often excised for the first level of a melanoma excision.[5] Some protocols excise the first level with a 5-mm clinical margin and then subsequent levels are excised by adding an additional 5 mm to positive margins.[2]

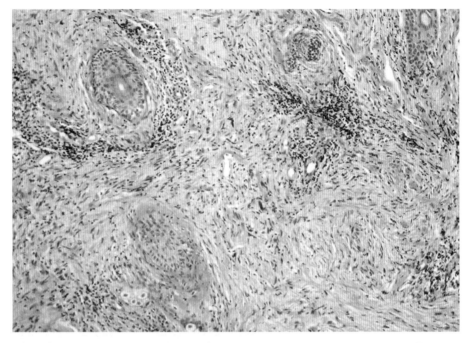

FIGURE 10.3. Invasive melanoma, desmoplastic type was found in the debulk specimen. The biopsy report in this case had revealed LM without invasion. Vertical sections of the debulk are needed to accurately diagnose the tumor and measure its thickness.

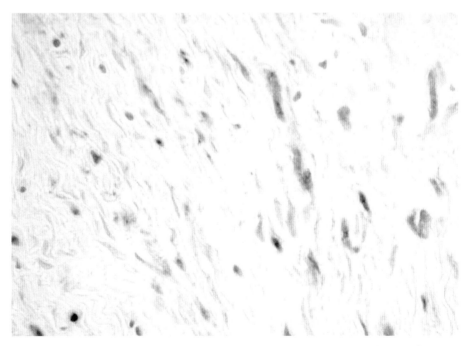

FIGURE 10.4. IHC with S100 can be needed to identify invasive desmoplastic melanoma. Other melanocytic IHC markers are frequently negative in this type of melanoma (e.g., Melan-A, HMB-45).

SPECIMEN PROCESSING TECHNIQUES

There is considerable overlap and therefore confusion in the terminology of the procedures. For the case of simplicity, it is helpful to consider the options as either **MMS**, which relies on the same frozen section pathology processes as MMS for other tumor types (described in Chaps. 3 and 6), or **modified MMS**, which is a paraffin section assessment.

MMS

After many years of dogma dictating that frozen sections should never be performed on melanoma specimens, it has now become well-established when examining the margins of LM. The relevant body of MMS literature is large, with many single-institution studies and occasional multi-institution studies demonstrating it to be an effective therapy, with low marginal recurrence rates and disease-specific survival rates comparable to—or better than—historical controls. The same processing principles as are used with MMS for other skin cancers apply, with the main difference being that the scalpel debulk step is essential for melanoma. IHC (usually with Melan-A, but sometimes with other markers) is often used as an adjunct.

Modified MMS

Modified MMS involves formalin-fixed, paraffin-embedded margin control in a team approach which separates the duties of the surgeon and pathologist.

Typically, the margins are removed and embedded *en face* in paraffin. Positive margins are mapped, and the patient returns for re-excision of any positive margins until the margins are proven to be negative, at which time reconstruction is performed. Variations arise from the shape of the excision (roundish or squarish) and whether the lesion with margin is excised by the surgeon as one unit *or* the surgeon removes just the margin as a strip before excising the whole lesion when negative radial margins are confirmed.

Johnson and colleagues described a modified MMS technique which has become known as the "square technique" (**Fig. 10.5**).[2,6] With this method, a double-bladed scalpel is used to remove the margin in strips in a square or rectangular shape around the melanoma. The square shape facilitates processing (laying the strip flat for embedding in paraffin) for examination of the entire margin. The first level is excised with a 5-mm margin around clinically visible tumor, with subsequent levels excised by adding an additional 5 mm to positive margins. The patient returns when the results of the margin assessment are known, and re-excision of the positive margin is repeated. A similar procedure but with a rounder shape has been referred to as the "spaghetti" or "linguine" technique.

A key point to remember with these various techniques is that the excision of the margins needs to be deep enough to ensure that the full thickness of hair follicles and adnexa are removed. This usually means excision to at least the mid-subcutaneous fat.

A major disadvantage to this process is the time required. Paraffin examination can be rapid, but never rapid enough to allow intraoperative assessment, so multiple days are usually needed to complete the procedure.

Hybrid Technique

Some teams prefer a technique which is best considered a combination of MMS and modified MMS. This involves excision with MMS frozen sections and, when the tumor is cleared, an additional safety margin is embedded *en face* in paraffin and examined (**Figs. 10.6** to **10.9**).

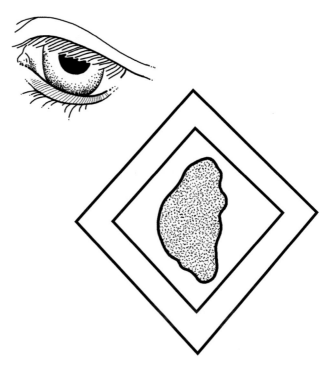

FIGURE 10.5. **In the "square technique," the radial margin is removed in a square strip around the melanoma.** When the radial margins have been clearer histologically, the central tumor is excised and the reconstruction is performed.

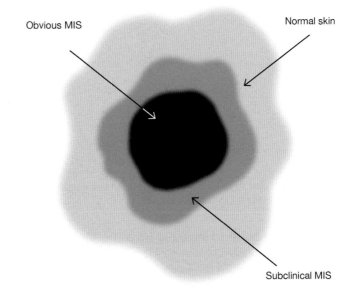

FIGURE 10.6. **In the hybrid technique, the clinical borders of any residual/remaining melanoma or biopsy scar are demarcated.** A dermatoscope and Wood's lamp examination can assist in this assessment.

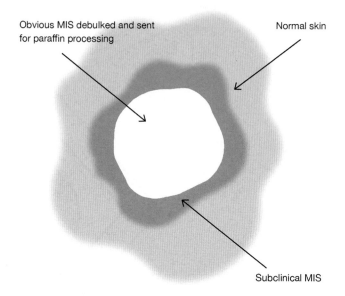

FIGURE 10.7. **The visible MIS is removed and sent for paraffin processing.** A margin of approximately 2 mm of normal-appearing skin is then excised as the first-stage margin. This must be excised to the deep subcutaneous fat to assure removal of the adnexal structures.

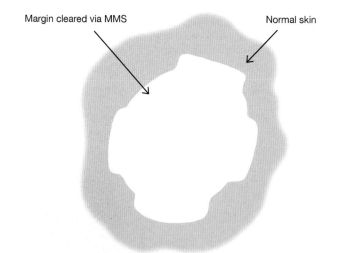

FIGURE 10.8. **Positive margins are mapped and additional margins of approximately 2 mm are taken in these areas until it is cleared.**

Management of Massive Invasive Melanoma

Large lesions of LM may have areas of deeply invasive LMM centrally. Though MCS is not recommended for deeply invasive melanoma, a caveat may be large in situ tumors on cosmetically sensitive skin with a central invasive tumor. In this scenario, MCS may be considered for the peripheral LM, in addition to complete excision and paraffin-embedded permanent section evaluation of the invasive disease. The central debulked tumor is bread-loafed and examined vertically to allow for accurate staging (**Figs. 10.10** to **10.13**).

Full "donut" sent to lab
to confirm clearance

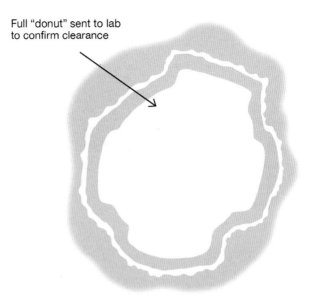

FIGURE 10.9. **Finally, following clearance of the lesion with frozen sections, an additional 2-mm safety margin is excised for paraffin processing.** If a complex reconstruction is needed, it is usually wise to keep the wound open until the negative margin is confirmed histologically. The safety margin in this context allows a thorough examination to check that nothing has been missed in the frozen section margin assessment. In difficult cases with extensive inflammation or actinic dysplasia, IHC can also be used on this specimen.

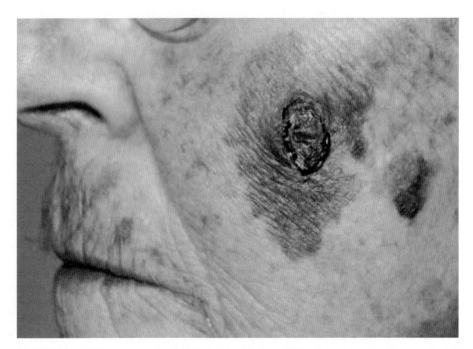

FIGURE 10.10. **MCS has a limited role in invasive melanoma.** This case presented with extensive LM with an invasive ulcerated tumor centrally. The central lesion was excised and sent for routine paraffin sections.

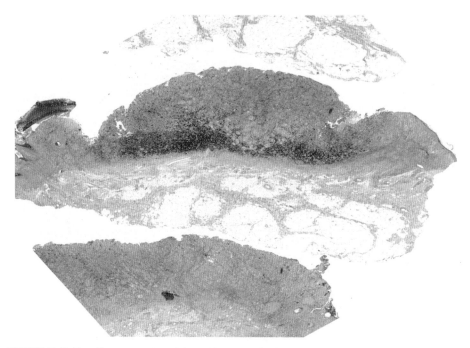

FIGURE 10.11. Paraffin assessment of the central invasive tumor was bread-loafed and examined vertically, allowing for assessment of the thickness of invasion, and other parameters for staging.

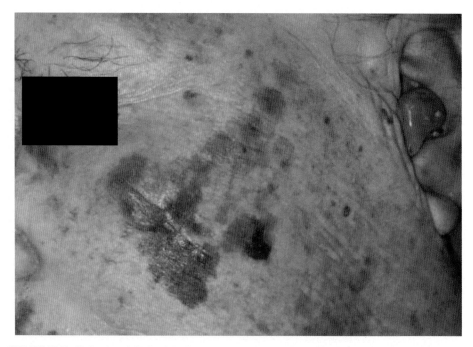

FIGURE 10.12. Following debulk of the invasive tumor, there was still extensive in situ disease present. Given the size of the tumor, the peripheral LM margins were assessed with intraoperative margin assessment using frozen sections.

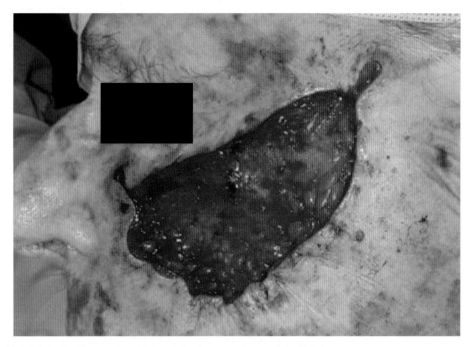

FIGURE 10.13. The resultant defect following complete excision is large.

"Mapped" Excision

Currently, most melanomas are still excised with WLE, and many continue to be processed by serial cross-sectioning (bread-loafing) of the tissue. When meticulous orientation is used with various colors recorded on a diagram, it is referred to as a "mapped" excision. Usually, the excision specimen is embedded in paraffin and sectioned vertically (bread-loafed as detailed in Chap. 6) at 1- to 3-mm intervals and entirely submitted for processing. Each block is step-sectioned to ensure thorough sampling. The wound is left open while the margin assessment is performed and the patient returns (often the next day) for further excision or repair as indicated.

A benefit of this method is the ability to measure the distance between the melanoma and the margin. A drawback is that the entire margin is not examined. To detect 100% of positive margins with this bread-loaf sectioning, Kimyai-Asadi et al. extrapolated that stepwise sections would need to be performed every 0.1 mm, which is not feasible.[6]

HISTOPATHOLOGY

LM is characterized histopathologically as a malignant melanocytic proliferation in the epidermis of sun-damaged skin. The melanocytes are arranged singly and often in nests and show nuclear hyperchromasia and pleomorphism. Melanocytes can be seen extending down adnexa and into the upper layers of the epidermis. In practice, LM includes a spectrum of morphologic changes ranging from low melanocyte cell density and a relatively bland cytology to more obvious malignant features such as high-cell density, disordered growth, and marked cytologic atypia. It can be very helpful to review the slides from a biopsy prior to surgery to gauge the expected features. The features are outlined in **Table 10.3** and **Figs. 10.14** to **10.20**.

TABLE 10.3 Main Histological Features of LM (**Figs. 10.14** to **10.20**)

- Proliferation of solitary and nested melanocytes at the dermal-epidermal junction
- Melanocyte cellular atypia (sometimes the atypia is subtle)
- Junctional nests of melanocytes in the epidermis of sun-damaged skin (with no dermal component)
- Melanocytes may extend into follicles and glands (**Fig. 10.16**)
- Starburst giant cells (multinucleated melanocytes) (**Fig. 10.17**)
- Associated lichenoid inflammatory reaction (**Fig. 10.18**)

The average number of melanocytes populating nonlesional skin of the head/neck skin is approximately 9 to 10 melanocytes per 0.5 mm. However, there are significant variations from patient to patient and there is overlap in cell density between the upper end of what can be "normal" and the lower end seen in LM. Rather than counting melanocytes per millimeter of epidermis, the impression of a discrete increase in melanocyte density above the background population over a stretch of skin is a more efficient way to quickly arrive at the correct diagnosis.[7]

In a recent analysis of factors involved in recurrence, the best features for distinguishing surrounding skin from the edge of LM included confluent growth, melanocyte density >15 per 0.5 mm, and adnexal spread. Normal skin may have runs of up to nine adjacent melanocytes with linear arrays of melanocytes extending along hair follicles, albeit without nesting or pagetoid spread.[8]

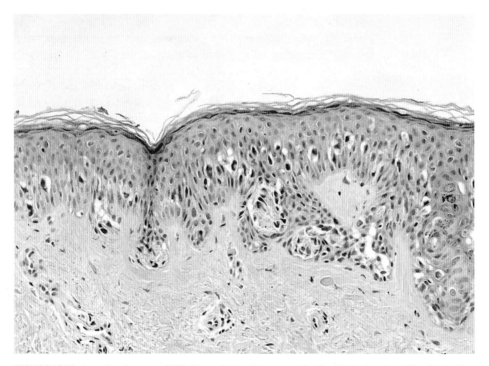

FIGURE 10.14. **In a classic case of LM, the melanocytes are markedly atypical and proliferate singly and in nests.** Also, there are malignant melanocytes in all levels of the epidermis (pagetoid extension) and extending down adnexal structures.

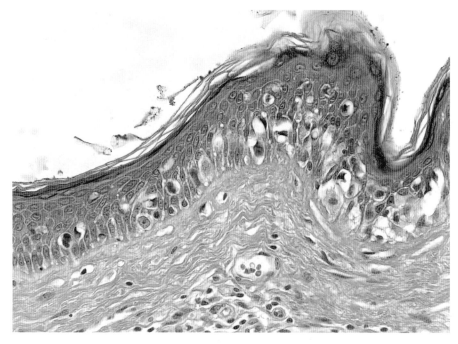

FIGURE 10.15. High-power examination shows there is a markedly atypical proliferation of melanocytes in the epidermis. The melanocytes are large, hyperchromatic, and proliferate irregularly in the epidermis. Some of the melanocytes are seen in the upper parts of the epidermis (pagetoid spread).

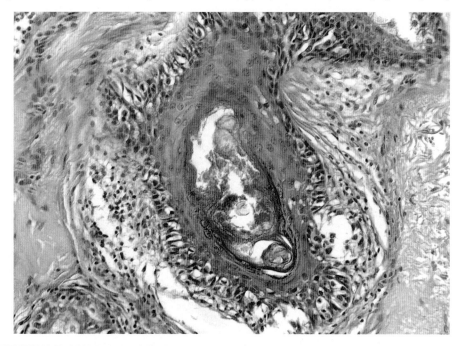

FIGURE 10.16. LM infiltrating follicular structures. This is common in LM, meaning careful examination of follicular structures is needed when assessing the radial margins. Excision down to at least mid-subcutaneous fat is needed to ensure the follicles are removed and examined.

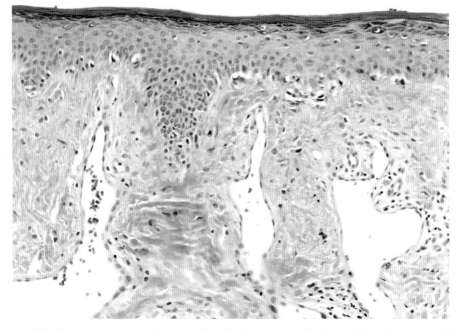

FIGURE 10.17. LM can sometimes be very subtle. Starburst giant cells (multinucleated melanocytes) as seen in the epidermis centrally in this photo can be a clue to subtle LM.

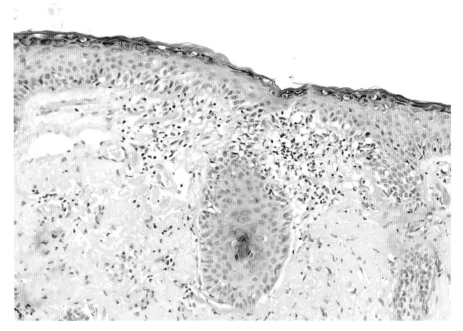

FIGURE 10.18. Lichenoid infiltrates can affect the epidermis and cause diagnostic confusion. Sometimes the collections of inflammatory cells resemble nests of melanocytes. Careful examination of the cellular morphology is needed to make the distinction. IHC is sometimes helpful.

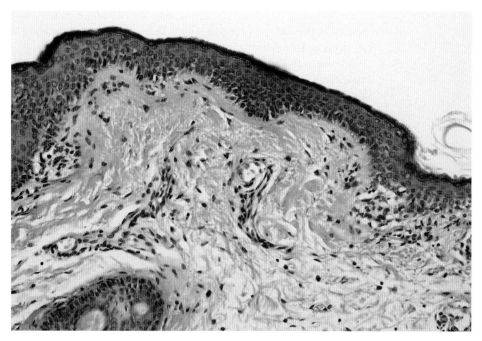

FIGURE 10.19. **LM has a spectrum of atypia.** In this example, small nests of melanocytes of LM are arranged irregularly along the epidermis. Though there is minimal nuclear atypia, the pattern of a junctional nested proliferation irregularly distributed on chronically sun-damaged skin of an elderly patient is consistent with LM.

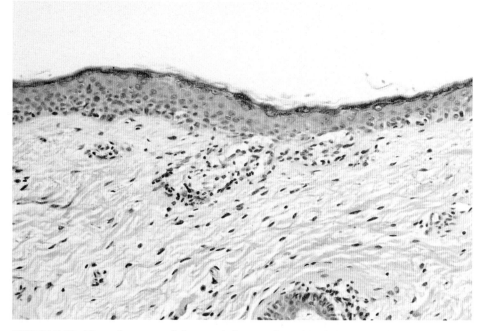

FIGURE 10.20. The melanocyte cellular morphology can be so bland that nests of melanocytes may be mistaken for collections of benign histiocytes.

Complicating the matters is actinic damage (dermatoheliosis), which can cause a mild increase in the number of melanocytes. These melanocytes can show striking atypia which can easily be mistaken for melanoma (**Fig. 10.21**).

Adding to this difficulty are artifactual changes in the frozen section slides which can cause keratinocytes and inflammatory cells to resemble melanoma. These artifacts can be minimized with careful attention to the freezing temperatures. The intermingling of melanoma cells with incidental actinic keratinocytic dysplasia is common and can also cause additional difficulties (**Fig. 10.22**).

IHC has become increasing popular for helping delineate melanocytic populations and avoiding potential pitfalls arising from artifacts. Rapid protocols have been developed and integrated into the workflow of intraoperative margin assessment. Melan-A is a very popular antibody for highlighting the native population of melanocytes (**Fig. 10.23**).

But IHC is not without its problems. A potential false-positive labeling for Melan-A may occur when the surgeon overestimates the extent of MIS and takes a wider margin than necessary. On sun-damaged skin, the melanocytes may show complex dendritic networks so that individual cells appear to be clusters of cells. Sox-10 is a nuclear stain which bypasses this problem (**Fig. 10.24**). There is also a limitation in sensitivity (some melanomas are negative for Melan-A), and occasional invasive melanomas may be missed by relying too much on IHC.

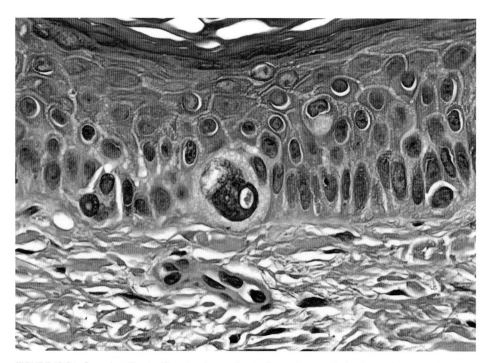

FIGURE 10.21. Occasionally, significant melanocytic atypia can be seen in benign melanocytes because of solar damage. These can easily be mistaken for melanoma. Key to interpretation is assessment of cellular density and the proximity to melanoma. (Image courtesy of Dr. Diego Morales, Philadelphia.)

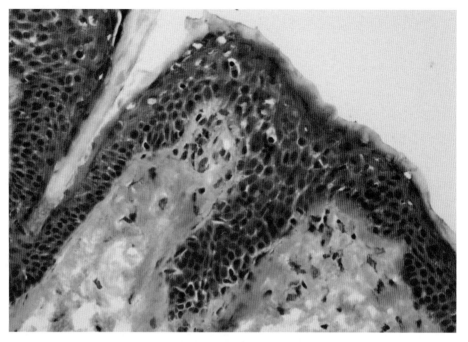

FIGURE 10.22. **Freezing can result in artifactual changes.** In this field, it is difficult to determine whether there is a melanocytic hyperplasia or inflammatory cells intermixed with the keratinocytes.

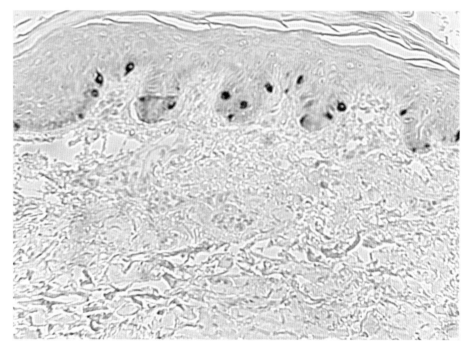

FIGURE 10.23. **IHC with Melan-A can be helpful in highlighting the population of melanocytes.** In this field, the melanocytes are evenly spaced. Features of concern include confluence of melanocytes, density of melanocytes >15 per 0.5 mm, spread down adnexal structures, and melanocyte nesting.

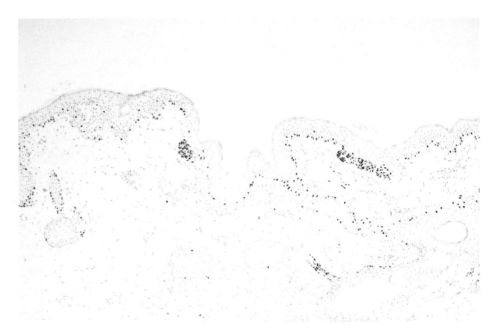

FIGURE 10.24. Sox-10 IHC stains the nucleus of melanocytes and highlights the nested proliferation of melanocytes in the epidermis in LM. Melan-A is more commonly used but is a cytoplasmic stain and interpretation can be challenging on sun-damaged skin.

Without a doubt, expertise in the interpretation of the slides is of critical importance. Some advocate for a multidisciplinary approach in which an independent dermatopathologist examines the rapid paraffin sections. Telepathology is a convenient way of accessing the expertise of a dermatopathologist intraoperatively. This method also allows the surgeon to view the slide together with the pathologist so that they can discuss the case and any issues surrounding interpretation and orientation.

SUMMARY

MCS is an attractive option for treating certain cases of melanoma. There are a few challenges, not least in defining the extent of the lesion clinically and in the interpretation of the histopathologic slides. But there is a range of procedural options to minimize these challenges and permit complete surgical excision with confidence.

References

1. National Comprehensive Cancer Network. Melanoma (Version1.2022). https://www.nccn.org/guidelines/guidelinesdetail?category=1&id=1430. Accessed December 17, 2021.
2. Swetter SM, Tsao H, Bichakjian CK, et al. Guidelines of care for the management of primary cutaneous melanoma. *J Am Acad Dermatol.* 2019;80(1):208-250.
3. Ellison PM, Zitelli JA, Brodland DG. Mohs micrographic surgery for melanoma: a prospective multicenter study. *J Am Acad Dermatol.* 2019;81(3):767-774.
4. Emanuel PO, Patel R, Zwi J, Cheng D, Izzard M. Utility of teledermatopathology for intraoperative margin assessment of melanoma in situ, lentigo maligna type: a 6 year community practice experience. *Eur J Surg Oncol.* 2021;47(5):1140-1144.

5. Thorpe RB, Covington KR, Caruso HG, et al. Development and validation of a nomogram incorporating gene expression profiling and clinical factors for accurate prediction of metastasis in patients with cutaneous melanoma following Mohs micrographic surgery. *J Am Acad Dermatol.* 2022;86(4):846-853.
6. Patel AN, Perkins W, Leach IH, Varma S. Johnson square procedure for lentigo maligna and lentigo maligna melanoma. *Clin Exp Dermatol.* 2014;39(5):570-576.
7. Kimyai-Asadi A, Katz T, Goldberg LH, et al. Margin involvement after the excision of melanoma in situ: the need for complete en face examination of the surgical margins. *Dermatol Surg.* 2007;33(12):1434-1439; discussion 1439-1441.
8. Star P, Rawson RV, Drummond M, Lo S, Scolyer RA, Guitera P. Lentigo maligna: defining margins and predictors of recurrence utilizing clinical, dermoscopic, confocal microscopy and histopathology features. *J Eur Acad Dermatol Venereol.* 2021;35(9):1811-1820.

11

Cutaneous Sarcomas

Patrick Emanuel / Mauricio León Rivera

General Considerations
AFX and PDS
DFSP
Cutaneous Leiomyosarcoma
Cutaneous Angiosarcoma

Common Mimickers of Sarcoma
    Nodular Fasciitis
    Keloid Scar
Summary

GENERAL CONSIDERATIONS

Cutaneous sarcomas are a diverse group of mesenchymal tumors arising in the dermis and subcutaneous tissues. Some are unique to this location while others represent the same tumor as is found in the deeper soft tissues. In general, superficial sarcomas have a better prognosis than their deeper counterparts.

Diagnosis is often challenging as these tumors are relatively rare. Frequently, the pathology needs to be reviewed by pathologists with significant experience in diagnosing sarcoma, which often means referral to the pathology department of a bone and soft tissue unit. The use of diagnostic immunohistochemistry (IHC) is required for practically all tumor types, and due to advancements in molecular pathology, diagnostic molecular techniques are frequently used.

With the possible exception for atypical fibroxanthoma (AFX), discussion at a multidisciplinary meeting (MDM) is almost always appropriate. There is a significant body of literature on many of these tumors that outlines the use of radiotherapy or systemic therapy, so this is the perfect forum to discuss these options.

Surgery is the definitive therapy and, since successful complete removal correlates with an improved outcome, a *complete* margin assessment is of particular benefit. Significant spread beyond what is evident clinically is a frequent feature. Once again it is worth emphasizing that margin control surgery (MCS) is the elimination of *guesswork*; wide local excision (WLE) following recommended margin sizes is *guessing* the actual size of the tumor. Unpredictability in the tumor's size means difficulty in both predicting surgical operating times and estimating the size of the resultant defect.

It is almost always appropriate to debulk the central tumor for paraffin assessment of the tumor parameters and confirmation of the diagnosis. This tissue can also be used for molecular analyses or research purposes.

Italian painters in the Renaissance period believed that no boundary in nature is sharply delineated and they developed the *sfumato* technique, which subtly blurred the transition between darker and lighter colors so that gradients could be reflected in their paintings. Somewhat similarly, aggressive sarcomas often have a histologic tumor border which melts into the surrounding normal tissue without a perceptible abrupt transition. In these cases, a precise histologic delineation of the tumor may be impossible, and a final wider paraffin safety margin may be needed.

The efficacy of MCS in treating some highly invasive sarcomas (e.g., angiosarcoma) is inconclusive in the literature. In this context, MCS may serve as a basic guide for the size and shape of the excision (see Chap. 6). This guidance is particularly helpful for tumors arising within a cosmetically or functionally sensitive anatomy.

AFX AND PDS

These tumors predominantly affect elderly patients with sun-damaged skin and have a predilection for the head and neck region, particularly the scalp. Clinically, they may present as a nodule or plaque, sometimes ulcerated, and often measure more than 2 cm (**Fig. 11.1**).

The prognosis is difficult to precisely define as many studies have lumped AFX together with pleomorphic dermal sarcoma (PDS). AFX generally has an excellent prognosis. In a large meta-analysis which encompassed a total of 914 cases of AFX, MCS showed a recurrence rate 2.0%, versus 8.7% without MCS, and metastatic disease was very rare.[1] In contrast, PDS has shown a local recurrence rate of 20% to 30% and a metastatic rate of 10% to 20%.[2]

Histologically, both AFX and PDS are characterized by a population of highly atypical mesenchymal cells which exhibit a wide-ranging morphology, from spindled cells to clear cells, as well as large epithelioid cells with multinucleated forms (**Figs. 11.2** and **11.3**).

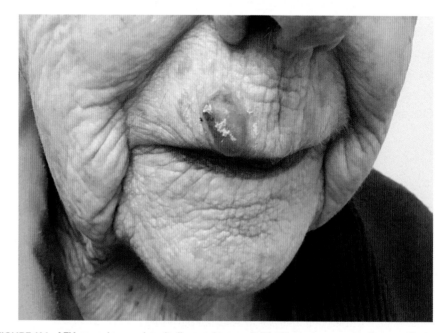

FIGURE 11.1. **AFX occurring on chronically sun-damaged skin.** These tumors are often exophytic, slow growing, and may resemble BCC clinically.

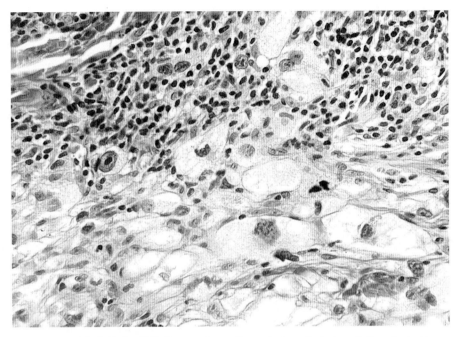

FIGURE 11.2. In this field, the AFX shows a clear cell morphology. Exclusion of other atypical tumors is needed when an unusual morphology is seen. AFX/PDS is negative with keratin markers which is helpful in excluding an unusual carcinoma.

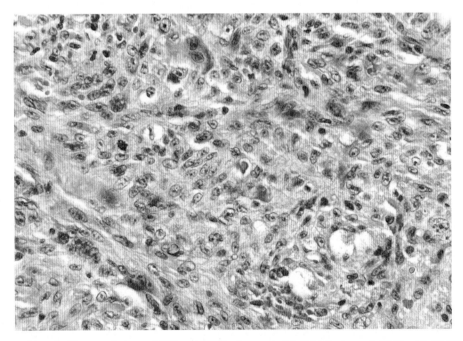

FIGURE 11.3. The morphology of AFX and PDS is diverse. In this field, the tumor is highly cellular and has an epithelioid to spindled morphology.

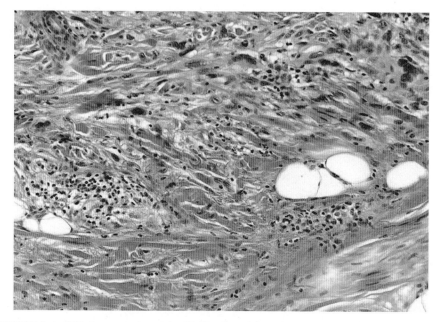

FIGURE 11.4. In AFX, there may be minimal infiltration of the subcutaneous fat. Extensive infiltration and infiltration of deeper structures (e.g., skeletal muscle, nerves) would suggest PDS rather than AFX. Some of these features only come to light at the time of MCS and need to be noted.

Due to this range, numerous histological variants have been reported, including desmoplastic, keloidal, granular, angiomatoid, hemosiderotic (pigmented), and myxoid variants. PDS is distinguished from AFX by identifying aggressive features: Extensive subcutaneous invasion, necrosis, and perineural or lymphovascular invasion are features to suggest PDS (**Fig. 11.4**).

The key feature is that these tumors are undifferentiated. Differentiation into a squamous, melanocytic, or distinct mesenchymal tissue (e.g., smooth muscle) is mutually exclusive to the diagnosis of AFX or PDS. Therefore, the histopathologic diagnosis is a diagnosis of exclusion and IHC is generally essential to rule out a high-grade carcinoma, an unusual melanoma, or other sarcoma (**Table 11.1**). Causing further difficulty, other sarcomas, melanoma, and poorly differentiated carcinoma can show areas which resemble AFX and PDS histologically. Careful attention always needs to be paid to looking for differentiation of another cell type. For example, thorough inspection of the overlying epidermis is required to look for evidence of *in situ* melanoma (**Figs. 11.5** and **11.6**).

TABLE 11.1 IHC for Cutaneous Sarcoma

	SOX-10, S100	CK5/6, p40	CD31	Desmin, SMA
AFX/PDS	Negative	Negative	Negative	Negative
SCC	Negative	Positive	Negative	Negative
Melanoma	Positive	Negative	Negative	Negative
Leiomyosarcoma	Negative	Negative	Negative	Positive
Angiosarcoma	Negative	Negative	Positive	Negative

SCC, squamous cell carcinoma.

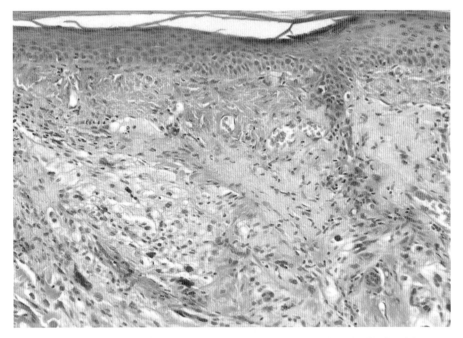

FIGURE 11.5. AFX is a dermally based tumor of highly atypical mesenchymal cells. Careful attention needs to be paid to the overlying epidermis. Melanoma in the overlying epidermis would point to the diagnosis of a sarcomatoid melanoma in the dermis rather than AFX.

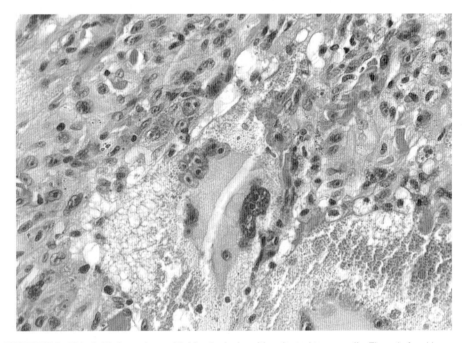

FIGURE 11.6. This field shows large, highly atypical multinucleated tumor cells. There is focal hae-mosiderin deposition which raises the possibility of melanin in melanoma.

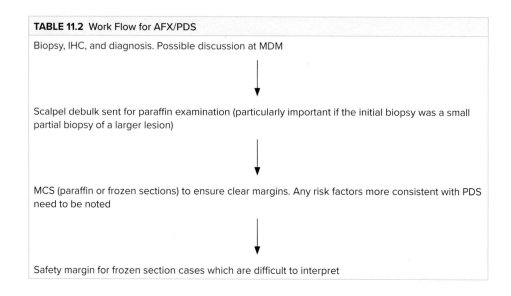

TABLE 11.2 Work Flow for AFX/PDS

Biopsy, IHC, and diagnosis. Possible discussion at MDM

↓

Scalpel debulk sent for paraffin examination (particularly important if the initial biopsy was a small partial biopsy of a larger lesion)

↓

MCS (paraffin or frozen sections) to ensure clear margins. Any risk factors more consistent with PDS need to be noted

↓

Safety margin for frozen section cases which are difficult to interpret

A common misconception is that CD10 is a specific immunohistochemical marker for AFX and PDS, but positivity may be seen in a wide range of tumors. A positive CD10 result is far less important than the exclusion of other diagnoses with IHC.

The cellular morphology is identical to the deep soft tissue tumor of malignant pleomorphic sarcoma (otherwise known as malignant fibrous histiocytoma or MFH) which—in contrast to AFX and PDS—is associated with a dismal prognosis.

Following confirmation of the diagnosis, MCS may be performed and uses the same principles as applied to skin carcinomas. The key difference comes in the careful attention that needs to be paid to the metrics which distinguish AFX from PDS. In the margin assessment sections, features of PDS may come to light: Extensive subcutaneous invasion, necrosis, and perineural or lymphovascular invasion would all need to be noted as these features would favor PDS. Cases of PDS may be referred to an MDM for consideration of radiotherapy or imaging studies.

In atypical cases with an unusual pathology (such as subtle histopathology or a pathology obfuscated by scarring from previous surgery), a safety margin for paraffin section examination as the final margin should be excised if possible.

The flow of the work is summarized in **Table 11.2**.

DFSP

Dermatofibrosarcom protuberans (DFSP) is a locally aggressive superficial mesenchymal neoplasm of fibroblastic derivation. It presents in a wide age range of patients with a median age at diagnosis between 20 and 69 years. Congenital and pediatric cases have also been described. It is usually a nodular, protuberant superficial mass. However, a diverse range of presentations has been described and the diagnosis is often a surprise. It frequently grows slowly for many years and sometimes then undergoes sudden progression.

Its tumorigenesis is associated with a translocation involving chromosomes 17 and 22, leading to the fusion of the collagen type 1alpha 1 (*COL1A1*) and platelet-derived growth factor subunit β (*PDGFB*) genes. This translocation results in a tyrosine kinase activation.

Tyrosine kinase inhibitors (e.g., imatinib mesylate) competitively inhibit ATP binding to the tyrosine kinase PDGF-beta receptor. This slows down kinase activity, limiting the growth of the tumor and promoting programmed cell death (apoptosis). This translocation can be demonstrated with cytogenetic testing (usually fluorescent in situ hybridization [FISH], see **Fig. 11.7**).

Complete surgical excision is the mainstay of treatment. While WLE (2-4 cm) was traditionally recommended, the NCCN currently recommends MCS for all cases of DFSP when possible (**Fig. 11.8**). The literature shows recurrence rates of approximately 1% for MCS, while WLE techniques have at times shown recurrence rates of over 20%.[3,4] Some surgical units still opt for the traditional wide excision, though in recent years, patients have increasingly become aware of the benefits of MCS (often through social media groups) and seek out providers who offer it.

Histopathologically, tumors are generally centered within the dermis or subcutis and are characterized by spindle cells with a storiform to whorled pattern. The cytoplasm is generally abundant and eosinophilic; the nuclei are monomorphic and ovoid to elongated with variable mitotic activity. The tumor infiltrates and expands fibrous septa; interdigitation among lobules of fat yields a so-called "honeycomb" pattern (**Figs. 11.9** and **11.10**).

Key to the diagnosis is positivity for CD34 with IHC. CD34 is positive in almost all cases (**Fig. 11.11**).

FIGURE 11.7. Fluorescent *in situ* hybridization (FISH) is a basic method for assessing *COL1A1-PDGFB* fusion, which is present in almost all cases of DFSP. Shown here is a dual color dual fusion probe (ZytoVision). In this, the *COL1A1* (17q21.33) is red and the *PDGF B* (22q13.1) is green. A positive result is indicated by a yellow signal (the red and green signals are fused together), implying a fusion of the *COL1A1-PDGFB* genes. (Image courtesy of Bernadette Garrone, Sullivan Nicolaides Pathology Cytogenetics, Australia.)

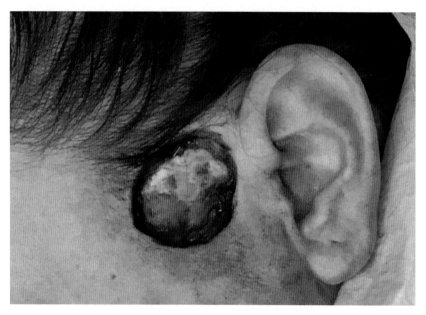

FIGURE 11.8. **This case of biopsy-proven DFSP had been excised with positive margins.** MCS with frozen sections allowed guidance for complete removal of what was clinically invisible residual tumor. The resulting defect following complete excision as seen here is quite modestly sized. A wide excision with *guessed* clinical margins may have resulted in a much larger excision. It is often impossible to know the extent of subclinical spread preoperatively, so guidance with MCS provides the best chance of complete removal with the best cosmetic result.

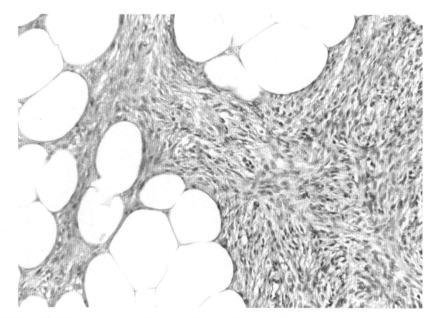

FIGURE 11.9. **DFSP is a spindle cell tumor infiltrating through adipose tissue with minimal intervening collagen.** In this example, the tumor is obvious but notice that the cellularity on the left of the image is decreased. In some areas, DFSP can be difficult to distinguish from fibrous tissue. CD34 IHC may be needed as DFSP is usually strongly positive.

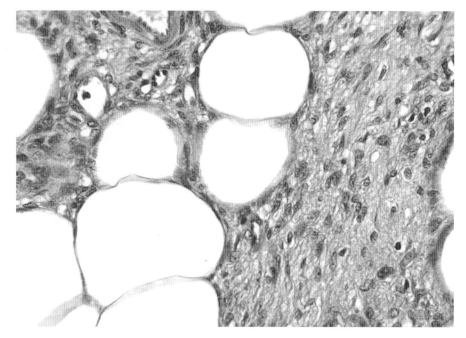

FIGURE 11.10. **High power highlights the spindle cell tumor.** The cytoplasm is abundant and eosinophilic; the nuclei are monomorphic and ovoid to elongated. Often very few mitoses are seen and there is little pleomorphism.

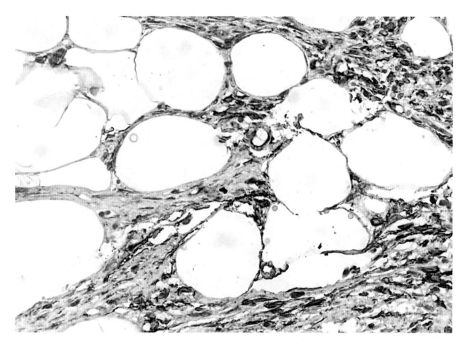

FIGURE 11.11. **IHC for CD34 can be helpful to define the margins histopathologically.** DFSP is generally diffusely positive. Care needs to be taken to be aware of background of normal dermal CD34 positivity. Examining the surrounding normal dermis, which serves as an internal control, is helpful.

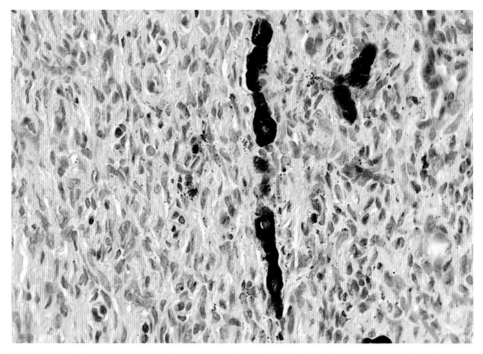

FIGURE 11.12. Bednar tumor is a distinctive rare form of DFSP which shows intermixed heavily pigmented spindled melanocytes.

Multiple variants exist, including those with giant cells[5] and melanin pigmentation (Bednar tumor)[6] (**Fig. 11.12**).

Fibrosarcomatous transformation has been reported to occur in 5% to 15% of DFSP and is thought to be associated with a higher rate of recurrence and metastasis. This transformation presents clinically as rapid enlargement, and histologically is characterized by a transformation into densely cellular spindle cell fascicles or a "herringbone" pattern with greater atypia and mitotic activity (**Fig. 11.13**).

The workflow for DFSP is summarized in **Table 11.3**.

CUTANEOUS LEIOMYOSARCOMA

Cutaneous leiomyosarcoma is a smooth muscle malignancy which typically presents as a rather nondescript slow-growing pink to purple skin tumor. When confined to the dermis, the prognosis is excellent and some authorities favor the term "atypical smooth muscle tumor" in this context (**Fig. 11.14**). The deeper form in the subcutis has a higher rate of recurrence and carries a small but definite risk for distant metastases. Rare cases are associated with immunodeficiency and EBV infection.

Histopathologically, mitotic figures (1/2 per 10 high-power fields), high cellularity, and bizarre myomatous cells are the generally accepted criteria for malignancy (**Figs. 11.15** and **11.16**). Smooth muscle differentiation can be illustrated with IHC for α-smooth muscle actin (α-SMA), muscle actin-specific (HHF35), and/or desmin.

The tumor is generally quite conspicuous histopathologically and tends to grow in a cohesive fashion. Subclinical growth can be extensive, with one series showing an average

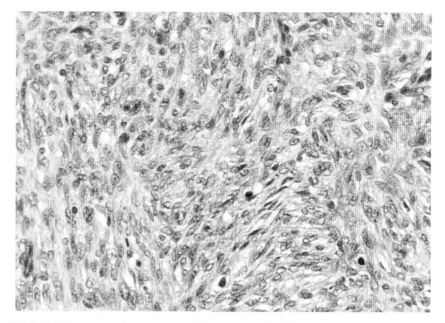

FIGURE 11.13. Fibrosarcomatous transformation is characterized by increased cellularity, greater atypia, and increased mitotic activity. It is important that special attention is paid to look for these changes during an MCS as these indicate a poorer prognosis, with an increased chance of recurrence and metastasis.

defect size of 15 cm following MCS. The evidence supporting MCS is strong, with a reported recurrence rate of 0% to 14% compared with the approximately 30% with WLE (0%-48% depending on the available follow-up data).[7]

TABLE 11.3 Workflow for DFSP

Biopsy for diagnosis. IHC with CD34. Cytogenetics for (*COL1A1-PDGFB*) may be performed. Discussion at MDM. Unresectable tumors may benefit from neoadjuvant therapy (oral tyrosine kinase inhibitor)

Scalpel debulk, particularly if the initial biopsy was small. This should be embedded in paraffin. Fibrosarcomatous differentiation may be encountered, which changes the prognosis

Margin assessment with MCS. CD34 may be used as an adjunct

Safety margin for paraffin sectioning and CD34 is often recommended to confirm negative margins, particularly in cases showing a highly infiltrative growth pattern

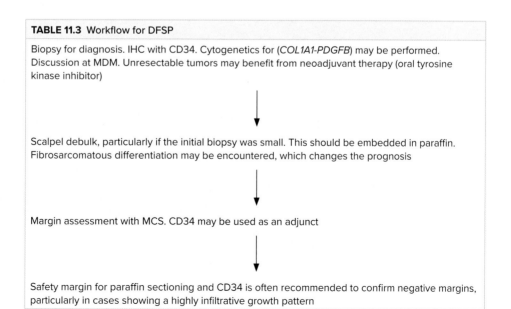

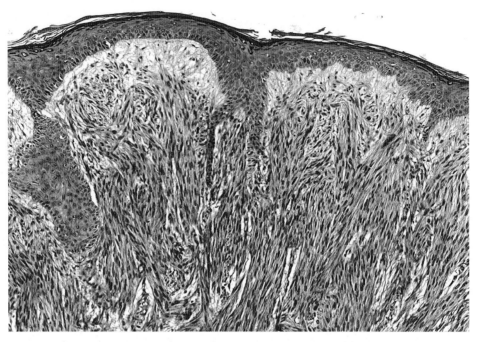

FIGURE 11.14. Cutaneous leiomyosarcoma often forms a dermal tumor underneath a normal epidermis. Superficial lesions have a much better prognosis than deeper tumors.

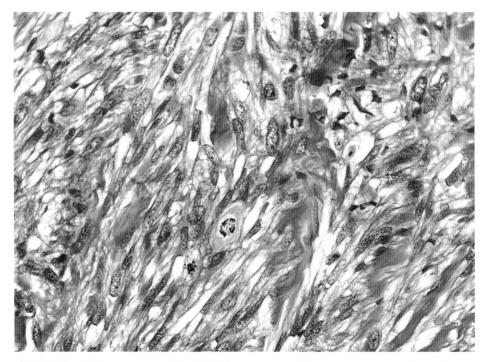

FIGURE 11.15. High-power examination highlights the atypia of the smooth muscle cells and the mitotic activity.

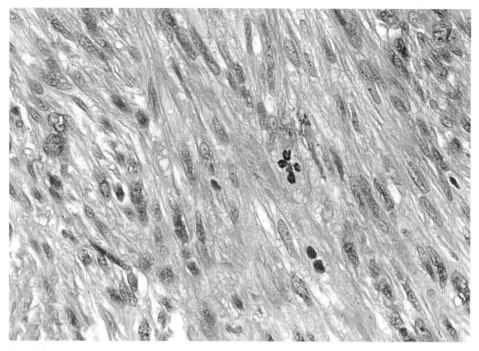

FIGURE 11.16. **The tumor is composed of cells with long nuclei with blunt ends ("cigar-shaped").** Distinction from leiomyoma is made by assessing pleomorphism and mitotic activity. In the field, we can see an X-shaped atypical mitosis which is generally not seen in benign leiomyoma.

CUTANEOUS ANGIOSARCOMA

Cutaneous angiosarcoma usually presents as a rapidly growing purple nodule or plaques (**Fig. 11.17**). There are three clinical contexts in which these arise: On the head and neck of the elderly, within chronic lymphedema, and following radiation (usually in the setting of breast cancer). Angiosarcoma is typically highly aggressive with frequent recurrence and metastasis.

Histologically, the tumor is a malignant neoplasm with vascular differentiation (**Figs. 11.18** and **11.19**). It has a broad histologic profile ranging from a well-differentiated neoplasm with frank vascular differentiation to a poorly differentiated tumor with epithelioid or spindled cells which can mimic AFX or another poorly differentiated malignancy. Its resemblance to AFX deserves special attention. In rare cases, vascular differentiation may only come to light at the time of MCS in treating angiosarcoma misdiagnosed as AFX. Therefore, it is important that an appropriate immunohistochemical panel has been ordered on a biopsy of AFX before MCS to ensure that the tumor is not actually an angiosarcoma.

IHC with CD31, ERG, FLI1, and MYC confirms a vascular origin. Some cases may be positive with cytokeratin stains which can cause diagnostic confusion. FISH studies show amplification of the *MYC* gene in most cases, so this may be performed in cases which are diagnostically challenging.

Given that surgery is the main therapeutic option for angiosarcoma, MCS may give some reassurance that the main bulk of the tumor is excised and can give guidance for

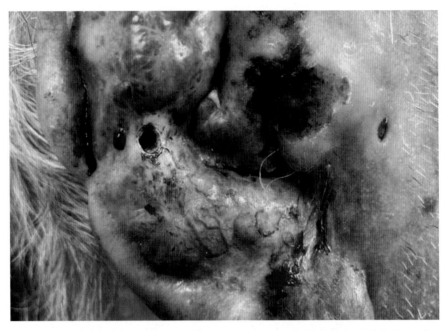

FIGURE 11.17. **Angiosarcomas are frequently fast-growing tumors with ill-defined clinical margins.** Given that surgery is the first-line therapy and the required surgery is often radical, MCS can offer some guidance to increase chances of a complete tumor removal. (Image courtesy of Dr. Henry Emanuel, Waikato Hospital, New Zealand.)

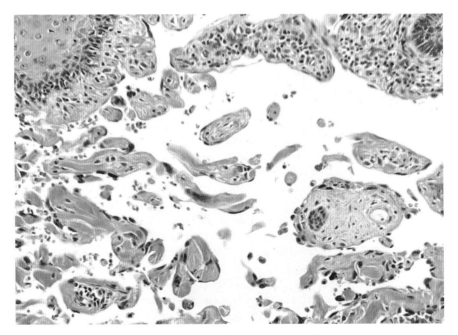

FIGURE 11.18. **In angiosarcoma, the malignant cells form vessels which often insinuate through the dermis and subcutis.** The lining cells of the vessels (endothelial cells) are hyperchromatic, pleomorphic, and large.

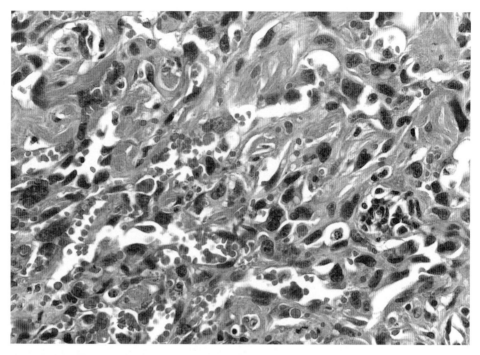

FIGURE 11.19. The vessels are poorly formed and lined by malignant endothelial cells. The presence of blood in the vascular spaces can be helpful in making the diagnosis.

large, poorly defined tumors requiring radical surgery. Use of a safety margin can provide further reassurance of negative margins but efficacy evidence is limited.

COMMON MIMICKERS OF SARCOMA

Nodular Fasciitis

This relatively common tumor can be mistaken for a sarcoma histologically, which is why it is mentioned here. It clinically presents as a fast-growing mass often on the limbs but also on the head and neck. It most commonly originates in the subcutis but in rare cases may arise in the dermis where it can cause diagnostic confusion. The histology is characteristic (**Fig. 11.20**): variable cellularity; extracellular matrix ranges from myxoid to collagenous; spindle stellate cells with a loose fascicular to storiform pattern (so-called "tissue culture-like" and "feathery" growth); scattered lymphocytes, histiocytes, and osteoclast type giant cells; and areas of extravasated erythrocytes.

Keloid Scar

Keloid scar may be mistaken for recurrence clinically. Thankfully, distinguishing keloid from sarcoma histologically is usually straightforward due to the identification of thick bands of collagen (**Fig. 11.21**). Rarely, keloid can be mistaken for malignancy histologically, particularly if the initial excision was for a sarcoma. Some areas of keloid exhibit high cellularity owing to the reactive proliferating myofibroblastic or fibroblastic cells showing nuclear enlargement and mitoses.

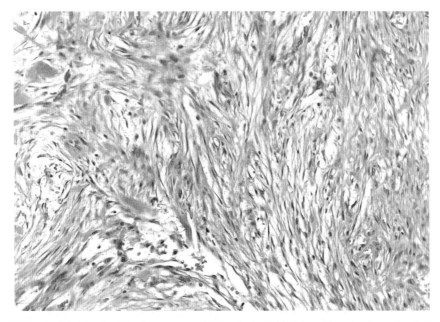

FIGURE 11.20. Nodular fasciitis shows a population of spindle stellate cells with a loose fascicular to storiform pattern (so-called "tissue culture" appearance). Helpful for the diagnosis is the presence of scattered lymphocytes and extravasated erythrocytes. The stroma may be keloidal (as seen focally here) or myxoid.

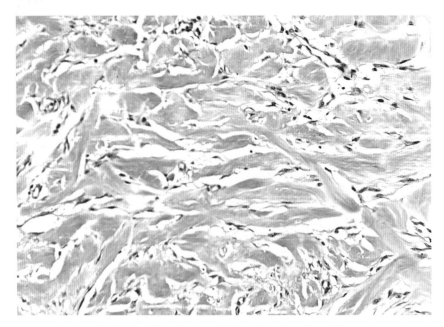

FIGURE 11.21. A keloid scar may result following previous surgery and can mimic a recurrence clinically, which is why it is shown here. In keloid, there are wide bands of collagen with large, brightly eosinophilic, glassy fibers. Between the collagen bundles, there are bland spindled fibroblasts and myofibroblasts.

SUMMARY

Cutaneous sarcomas are histologically diverse and can be diagnostically challenging. The use of diagnostic pathology techniques aids in defining these tumors. Most are readily seen in frozen sections, so intraoperative MCS is an excellent option that avoids *guesswork*.

References

1. Tolkachjov SN, Kelley BF, Alahdab F, Erwin PJ, Brewer JD. Atypical fibroxanthoma: systematic review and meta-analysis of treatment with Mohs micrographic surgery or excision. *J Am Acad Dermatol.* 2018;79(5):929-934.e6.

2. Miller K, Goodlad JR, Brenn T. Pleomorphic dermal sarcoma: adverse histologic features predict aggressive behavior and allow distinction from atypical fibroxanthoma. *Am J Surg Pathol.* 2012;36(9):1317-1326.

3. Paradisi A, Abeni D, Rusciani A, et al. Dermatofibrosarcoma protuberans: wide local excision vs. Mohs micrographic surgery. *Cancer Treat Rev.* 2008;34:728-736.

4. Matin RN, Acland KM, Williams HC. Is Mohs micrographic surgery more effective than wide local excision for treatment of dermatofibrosarcoma protuberans in reducing risk of local recurrence? A critically appraised topic. *Br J Dermatol.* 2012;167:6-9.

5. Beham A, Fletcher CD. Dermatofibrosarcoma protuberans with areas resembling giant cell fibroblastoma: report of two cases. *Histopathology.* 1990;17(2):165-167.

6. Dupree WB, Langloss JM, Weiss SW. Pigmented dermatofibrosarcoma protuberans (Bednar tumor). A pathologic, ultrastructural, and immunohistochemical study. *Am J Surg Pathol.* 1985;9(9):630-639.

7. Starling J 3rd, Coldiron BM. Mohs micrographic surgery for the treatment of cutaneous leiomyosarcoma. *J Am Acad Dermatol.* 2011;64(6):1119-1122.

12

Merkel Cell Carcinoma

Patrick Emanuel / Mark Izzard

Examination
Surgical Management Strategies
   Less-Advanced Tumors
   More-Advanced Tumors

Histopathology
Histopathologic Differential Diagnosis
Summary

Merkel cell carcinoma (MCC) is an aggressive neuroendocrine carcinoma of the skin with high rates of metastasis and death. It was first described by Cyril Toker in 1972 who called it trabecular carcinoma. Later, it was named after the Merkel cells (specialized pressure receptor cells in the epidermis) as these are histologically and immunophenotypically like MCC tumor cells. MCC is most common in the 7th to 9th decades of life and frequently arises on chronically sun-exposed skin of the head and neck (>40%). Immunosuppression is also a risk factor with higher rates in patients with hematological malignancy, HIV, and iatrogenic immunosuppression.

Development of MCC follows two distinct pathways: Infection with the Merkel cell polyomavirus (approximately 80% of cases but this varies geographically), *or* somatic mutations caused by chronic UV exposure. The distinct pathogenic pathways have led some authors to believe that MCC represents two distinct entities based on their etiology. The cell of origin may be keratinocytes, fibroblasts, or B lymphocytes rather than native Merkel cells.

Surgical excision is the first-line treatment, yet there is no clear consensus on the size of the excision margin.

EXAMINATION

MCC grows as a painless nodular lesion, with a blue or red tinge. Typically, it presents abruptly and explodes into a rapidly growing tumor (**Fig. 12.1**). Other rapidly growing dermal tumors are in the clinical differential such as lymphoma, amelanotic melanoma, metastatic disease, or sarcoma.

Heath et al. introduced the helpful mnemonic AEIOU as an aide to the clinical diagnosis[1]: Asymptomatic, Expanding rapidly, Immunosuppression, Older than 50, UV exposed site.

Nodal disease is seen in up to 80% of head and neck cases at presentation. Checking clinically for nodes at the time of examination can be a helpful differentiator from basal cell carcinoma (BCC). Generally, MCC patients should undergo a staging PET/CT scan.

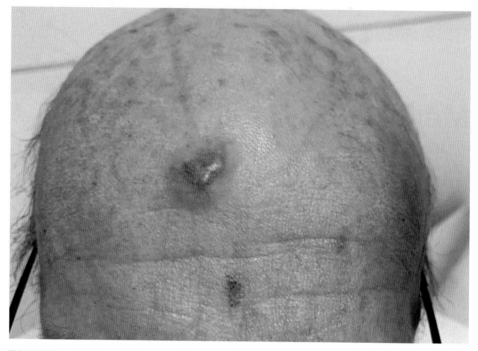

FIGURE 12.1. **MCC presents as a rapidly enlarging dermal mass.**

Presentation at a multidisciplinary meeting (MDM) to discuss treatment options prior to surgery is also prudent.

SURGICAL MANAGEMENT STRATEGIES

Complete surgical excision is the therapy of choice, and margin control surgery (MCS) can guide the extent of the excision. All patients with resectable disease and who are fit for surgery may be offered one of the two following plans:

Less-Advanced Tumors
MCS of primary MCC under local anesthetic.

If the lesion turns out to be small, the wound can be reconstructed on the same day under local anesthetic. MCC MCS often requires multiple levels and may take all day to get an adequate radial clearance, so general anesthetic is not ideal. However, if it turns out intraoperatively that the MCC is deeply invasive (e.g., with invasion of structures such as the skull, parotid, or nerves), initial clearance of at least peripheral margins under local anesthetic may be performed, and then a general anesthetic (often at a later date) is needed for resection of deeper structures such as the parotid gland or regional lymph nodes (**Figs. 12.2** to **12.4**).

More-Advanced Tumors
Multiple levels are anticipated, and a neck dissection and/or a complex reconstruction are to be done in the same session under general anesthetic.

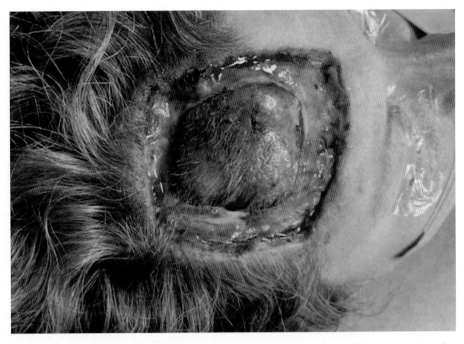

FIGURE 12.2. **The deep margin of this MCC abutted the skull.** The peripheral margin was cleared under local anesthetic with frozen sections. A safety margin was processed in paraffin. Note the discoloration due to vascular compromise.

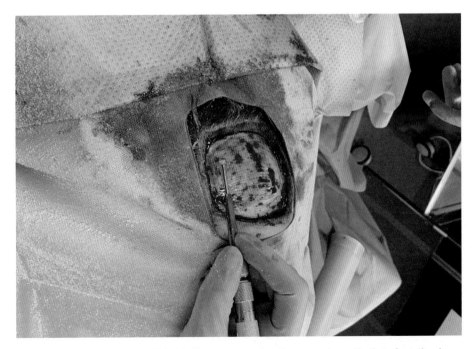

FIGURE 12.3. The outer table of the skull was removed under general anesthetic to form the deep margin.

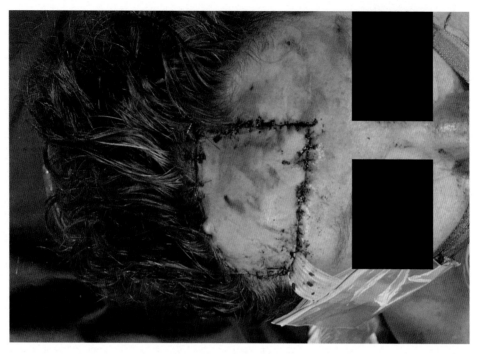

FIGURE 12.4. Reconstruction was performed under general anesthesia in the same session as the outer table resection.

Even if the primary tumor can be cleared under local anesthetic, if the patient needs a neck dissection or extensive reconstruction, general anesthesia will generally be needed.

In this scenario, the patient is put to sleep and the first level is removed and processed. The primary site is then shut off, a clean re-drape is done, and a clean surgical set is used to perform the neck dissection while the surgeon waits for the level of the skin to be processed.

For areas that cannot be assessed with frozen sections such as skull or facial bones, it is best to operate to the anatomy. Examples include removing the outer table of the skull (**Fig. 12.3**), or segmental mandibulectomy, followed by reconstruction of the missing unit.

A final safety margin processed in paraffin can help to assure that the final margin is negative, regardless of the method chosen.

HISTOPATHOLOGY

The histopathology of MCC can range from being readily recognizable to being quite difficult and subtle. The biopsy should be reviewed. A general idea of the tumor morphology prior to surgery can thus be obtained, and this ensures that adequate immunohistochemistry (IHC) has been performed and that other possibilities can be excluded (**Table 12.1**). Morphologically, the tumor cells have almost no cytoplasm and round/oval nuclei. The chromatin in the nuclei is characteristic of a finely dispersed grainy quality often described as "salt and pepper" (**Fig. 12.5**).

TABLE 12.1 IHC for MCC and Its Differential Diagnosis

Tumor	Basic Morphology	IHC
MCC	Neuroendocrine (salt and pepper chromatin). Small round blue cells	CK20+, neurofilament+, TTF1−, chromogranin+, synaptophysin+
BCC	Basaloid, peripheral palisading, retraction artifact	CK20−, neurofilament−, TTF1−, chromogranin+/−, synaptophysin+/−
Metastatic neuroendocrine carcinoma (small cell carcinoma)	Neuroendocrine (salt and pepper chromatin). Small round blue cells	CK20−, neurofilament−, TTF1+, chromogranin+, synaptophysin+
Lymphoma	Lymphoid cells	Leukocytic common antigen+

Three histopathologic patterns may be seen (**Figs. 12.5** to **12.8**): The small cell type has solid sheets and clusters of cells which are small, round, and often mimic a lymphoma; the trabecular type has cells arranged in interconnected trabeculae separated by strands of stromal tissue; and the intermediate cell type has cells arranged in large nests. Co-occurrence with squamous cell carcinoma (SCC) is not uncommon and this needs to be kept in mind when examining SCC resections (an incidental diagnosis of MCC radically changes the

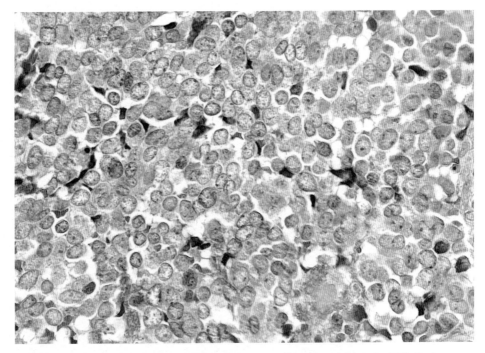

FIGURE 12.5. MCC may grow in solid sheets and nests, and may be mistaken for BCC. Key to distinction is the nuclear detail. In MCC, the cells have almost no cytoplasm and have round/oval nuclei. The chromatin on the nuclei is finely dispersed and often described as "salt and pepper." This morphology of MCC is easy to see in frozen section slides.

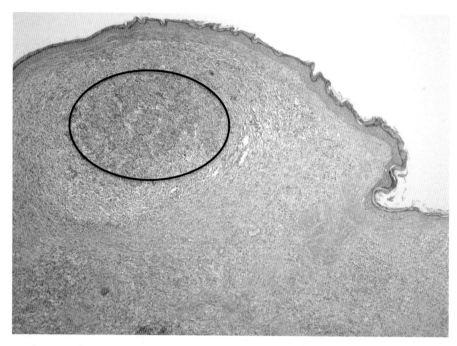

FIGURE 12.6. MCC may at times look more like a lymphoma or an inflammatory process. In this example, the focus of MCC could easily be overlooked in the profusion of chronic inflammatory changes. This is an example of the small cell morphology of MCC.

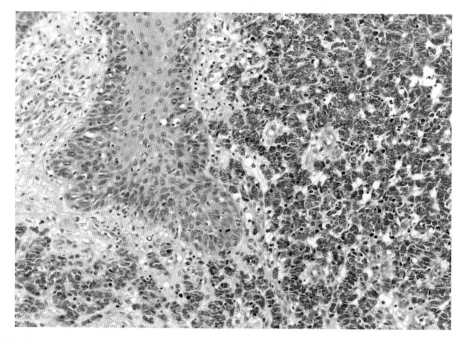

FIGURE 12.7. MCC is frequently seen intermixed with SCC. In this example, we can see there is dysplasia of the basal epidermis. This MCC shows a trabecular pattern in areas. MCC can rarely be found in frozen section slides for excision of SCC.

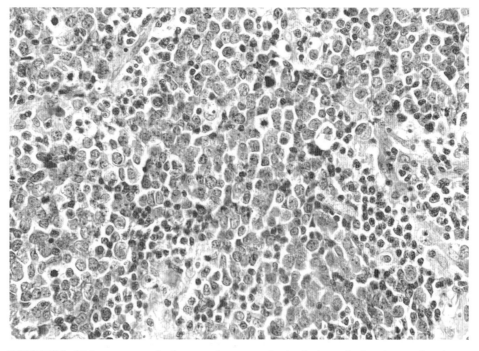

FIGURE 12.8. **High-power examination reveals neuroendocrine features: "salt and pepper" grainy chromatin with numerous mitoses and marked atypia.** This is an example of the intermediate cell morphology of MCC. We can also see an admixed population of small clonal lymphocytes consistent with chronic lymphocytic lymphoma. Hematologic diseases are a risk factor for MCC.

prognosis). Co-occurrence with lymphoma may also be seen. In unusual cases, differentiation to other cell types occurs, such as melanocytic, eccrine, leiomyosarcomatous, rhabdomyoblastic, or fibrosarcomatous differentiation.

HISTOPATHOLOGIC DIFFERENTIAL DIAGNOSIS

When extensive satellite growth is seen, it raises the possibility of neuroendocrine carcinoma metastatic from another site such as small cell carcinoma of the lung, which can be histologically identical. IHC can help (**Table 12.1**), but sometimes even that is not reliable and radiologic correlation may be needed to completely exclude metastasis from the lung.

With IHC, MCC shows a typical perinuclear dot pattern with CK20 in a high proportion of cases (**Fig. 12.9**) as well as neurofilament positivity in almost all cases (**Fig. 12.10**).

When MCC grows in a nodular fashion, it can be misdiagnosed as a BCC if careful attention is not paid at high-power magnification. MCS may begin as an excision of a BCC but change to an MCC procedure if the previous biopsy has been misdiagnosed. Another significant challenge is that the nuclei of MCC cells have an extremely high DNA concentration, meaning that they can be crushed during processing and thus resemble inflammatory cells (**Fig.12.11**).

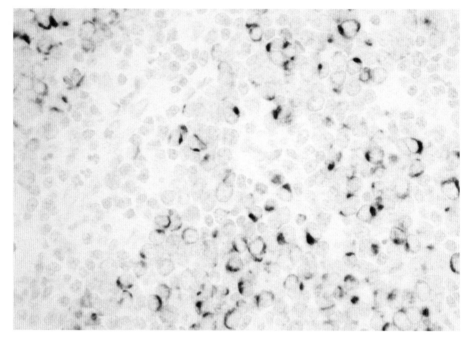

FIGURE 12.9. IHC can aid in the diagnosis and in assessing the margins, particularly when the morphology is unusual. MCC will be positive with CK20 in this characteristic perinuclear pattern.

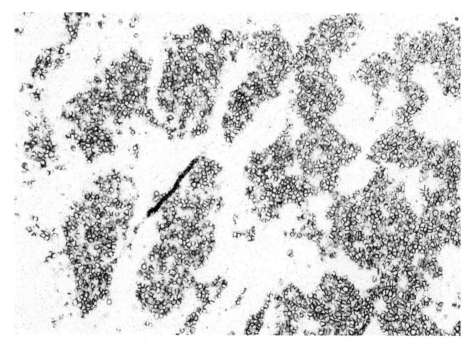

FIGURE 12.10. Other stains such as the neuroendocrine markers (chromogranin, synaptophysin) will also be positive. A percentage of MCC (up to 10%) will be negative with CK20. In these cases, neurofilament can be helpful as almost all MCC is positive with this marker, as shown in this image.

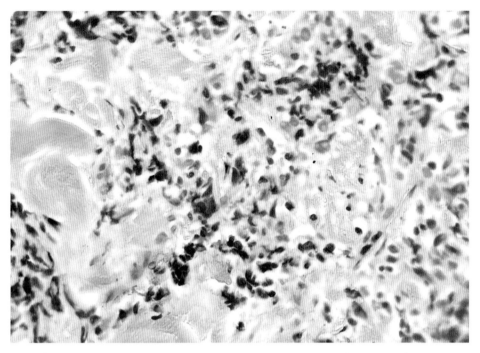

FIGURE 12.11. **The malignant cells may be crushed during processing and resemble inflammatory cells.** Examination of surrounding intact areas can be helpful. It is generally advised to err on the side of caution with MCC and to regard suspicious areas as likely to be positive.

SUMMARY

MCC can be a challenging tumor to deal with due to its aggressive clinical course as well as its varied histopathology, which may be mistaken for another more common malignancy. Correct diagnosis, clinical planning, and appreciation of the histopathologic subtleties are all key to successful MCS.

Reference

1. Heath M, Jaimes N, Lemos B, et al. Clinical characteristics of Merkel cell carcinoma at diagnosis in 195 patients: the AEIOU features. *J Am Acad Dermatol.* 2008;58(3):375-381.

13

Malignant Adnexal Tumors

Patrick Emanuel / Mark Izzard

General Considerations
    Biopsy
    Debulk
    Mapping
    Safety Margin
Specific Tumor Types
    MAC
    Differential Diagnosis for MAC
    Porocarcinoma

Hidradenocarcinoma
Sebaceous Carcinoma
Eccrine Spiradenocarcinoma
EMPSGC
Primary Mucinous Carcinoma of the Skin
Adenoid Cystic Carcinoma
ADPA
PHCE
Summary

From the Latin *adnexa* meaning attached or conjoined, *adnexal* refers to the appendages of organs, in this case, of the skin. The large heterogenous group of malignancies arising from these appendages can represent both diagnostic and surgical management difficulties.

GENERAL CONSIDERATIONS

Clinically, these tumors are rather nondescript, presenting as enlarging dermal tumors. Some malignant adnexal tumors grow within their benign counterparts so a common presentation is recent growth in a long-standing tumor.

Surgery is the mainstay of treatment. Due to an infiltrative growth pattern, these tumors often extend more widely than is appreciated clinically so surgical plans can radically change intraoperatively. Most arise on the head and neck where tissue preservation is frequently a key concern.

Successful margin control surgery (MCS) is dependent on an accurate biopsy diagnosis and the ability to identify and track the tumor with frozen section examination. It is helpful to prepare the patient and the staff for the possibility of multiple levels, a long day, and a sizeable defect. A multistage procedure is often planned with a delayed reconstruction. The usual workflow is outlined in **Table 13.1**.

Biopsy

Given the rarity of some of these tumors, review of the biopsy is generally advisable. If the biopsy is not available for review, an onsite biopsy is recommended. The biopsy needs to demonstrate the way in which the tumor interacts with surrounding tissues, so a deep incisional biopsy is generally preferred. Correlating the histologic diagnosis with the clinical

TABLE 13.1 Usual Workflow

(i) Biopsy review, IHC, and diagnosis. Possible discussion in the multidisciplinary meeting (MDM)
(ii) Central debulk sent for paraffin assessment
(iii) MCS (paraffin or frozen section) to ensure clear margins. Be prepared for multiple levels, complex mapping, and chasing perineural invasion
(iv) Paraffin safety margin should be considered for difficult FS cases
(v) Consider delayed reconstruction after safety margin assessment

findings can be critical. For example, plaque-type syringoma is generally obvious clinically, but it may be misdiagnosed pathologically as microcystic adnexal carcinoma (MAC); MCS in this context (the unnecessary complete excision of a large benign syringoma) can have disastrous cosmetic and functional consequences.

Debulk
The central tumor is debulked and sent for formal histology to confirm the diagnosis and check for risk factors (e.g., perineural invasion) which may not be evident on the initial biopsy. This tissue may also be used for further studies (diagnostic, therapeutic, or research).

Mapping
Often the lesion is large, so a meticulous surgical diagram of serial blocking is important. The following figures demonstrate a typical difficult case (**Figs. 13.1** to **13.4**).

Safety Margin
For subtle or aggressive tumors, it may be sensible to extend the final margin with a paraffin safety margin.

SPECIFIC TUMOR TYPES

MCS has been shown to be a useful therapy for a vast array of adnexal carcinomas but the full range of these tumors is beyond the scope of this chapter. Emphasis will be given to tumors which have been given the most attention in the literature and in which the authors have specific experience.

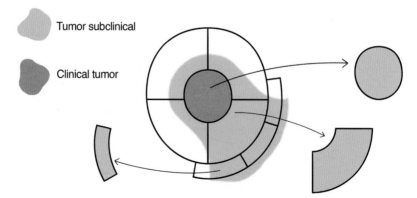

FIGURE 13.1. **The clinical tumor is debulked and sent to the laboratory for paraffin sectioning.** The entire peripheral and deep margin is removed, mapped, and examined *en face*.

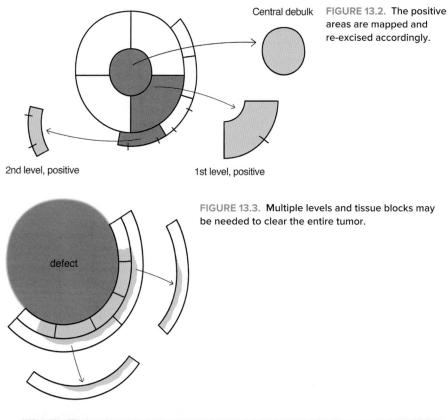

Central debulk

FIGURE 13.2. The positive areas are mapped and re-excised accordingly.

2nd level, positive

1st level, positive

FIGURE 13.3. Multiple levels and tissue blocks may be needed to clear the entire tumor.

defect

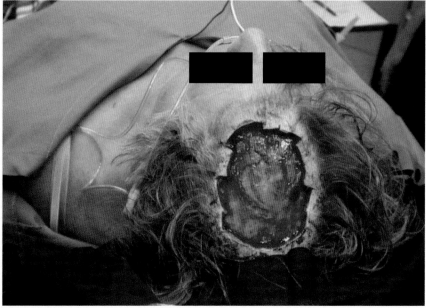

FIGURE 13.4. Some cases of MAC can result in a large defect. This example was much larger than initially anticipated.

MAC

MAC is a sweat gland carcinoma which is thought to originate from an adnexal keratinocyte capable of undergoing follicular or sweat gland differentiation. It typically presents as a slow-growing nodule or scar-like plaque on the lip or face. Neurological symptoms such as numbness and tingling are common due to perineural invasion. MAC frequently extends well beyond the clinically estimated extent. Resultant surgical defects following MCS have been shown to be four times larger than preoperative estimates.[1,2] MRI may be helpful to delineate the extent of disease preoperatively. On rare occasions, advanced cases may benefit from neoadjuvant radiotherapy before surgery. Unprotected sun exposure and previous radiation therapy are known risk factors.

Though metastasis is uncommon, recurrence is common and can be destructive. The literature suggests MCS has a favorable recurrence rate when compared with wide local excision (WLE). With five years of follow-up, the rate of recurrence following MCS ranges from 0% to 22%, while recurrence rates for WLE approach 50%.[1]

Histopathologic misdiagnosis of the biopsy is common, and the correct diagnosis of MAC is only made in the first instance during MCS in up to 32.5% of cases.[2] It is, therefore, important to understand the pathology of MAC and the common differential diagnoses.

Histopathologically, MAC is an infiltrative tumor based in the dermis (**Fig. 13.5**) and usually invades subcutaneous tissues (**Fig. 13.6**). The tumor is composed of squamous islands and thin cords with areas of ductal (glandular) differentiation. Superficially, keratinous cysts may be seen. The intervening stroma may be sclerotic. Commonly, small nerves are invaded (**Fig. 13.7**).

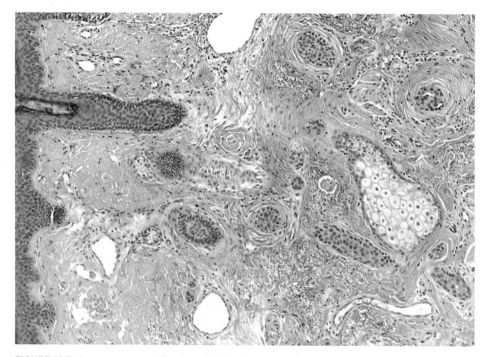

FIGURE 13.5. Low-power magnification of MAC shows cords and nests composed of quite bland tumor cells invading the full thickness of the dermis and into subcutis.

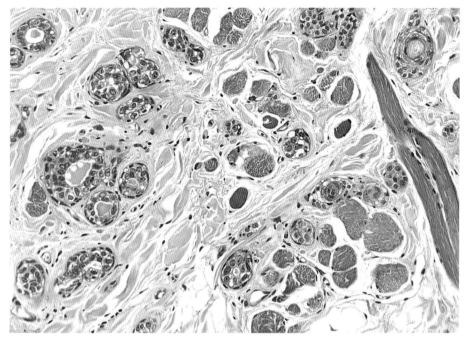

FIGURE 13.6. **At higher-power examination of MAC, the ductal (glandular differentiation) can be appreciated.** Small islands and strands of epithelial cells infiltrate deeply through the skeletal muscle. The cells are deceptively bland with minimal cytologic atypia and only rare mitotic figures.

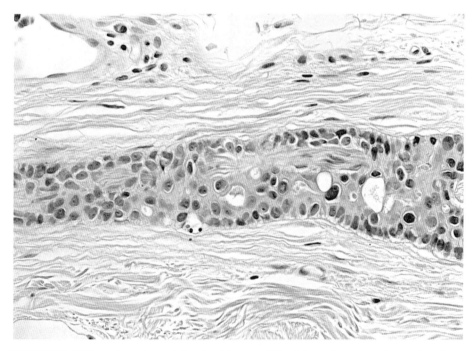

FIGURE 13.7. **MAC can be seen encasing a small nerve.** Often this can be seen well away from the main tumor mass.

Differential Diagnosis for MAC

A confident diagnosis of MAC can be impossible with limited material such as a small superficial shave biopsy. The superficial features may almost precisely mimic sclerosing tumors such as desmoplastic trichoepithelioma (**Fig. 13.8**), infiltrative BCC (**Fig. 13.9**), and syringoma (**Fig. 13.10**). Unfortunately, immunohistochemistry (IHC) continues to have only a limited role in the distinction. A deep biopsy (to subcutis is preferred) to demonstrate the association of the tumor with the subcutis and nerves as well as to see evidence of an infiltrative pattern through the dermis is often needed. The histopathologic differential diagnosis is summarized in **Table 13.2**.

The high rate of recurrence may also be attributed to the subtle histopathology which can be overlooked, particularly in the case of small foci of perineural invasion at the surgical margin. A safety margin sent in paraffin is useful to delineate the extent of the margin positivity in the final stage. IHC for cytokeratin can be helpful in delineating subtle perineural invasion.

Porocarcinoma

Porocarcinoma (or eccrine porocarcinoma) arises from the dermal sweat gland duct and the acrosyringium. It arises either *de novo* or from preexisting benign eccrine poroma (approximately 20% of cases) and presents clinically as nodular, infiltrative, ulcerated, or polypoid growths most commonly on the extremeties. According to the literature,

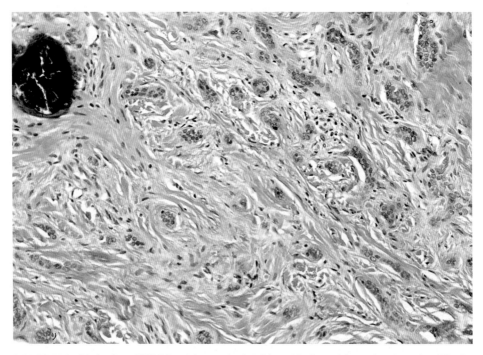

FIGURE 13.8. Distinction of MAC from desmoplastic trichoepithelioma (shown here) can be difficult. Desmoplastic trichoepithelioma does not display ductal (glandular) differentiation. The tumor has small islands of basaloid epithelium superficially which form cords and strands toward the base and periphery. Superficially, MAC also often lacks glandular differentiation which is why it may be impossible for superficial biopsies to facilitate distinction.

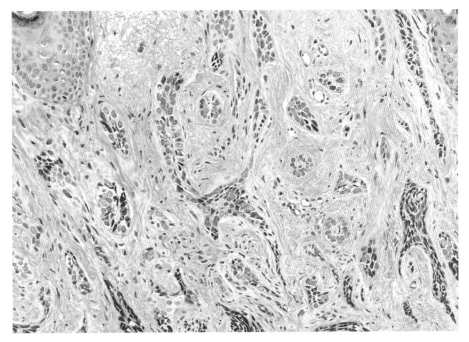

FIGURE 13.9. Infiltrative BCC is a variant of BCC characterized by narrow strands and nests of basaloid cells. The glandular differentiation characteristic of MAC is not seen.

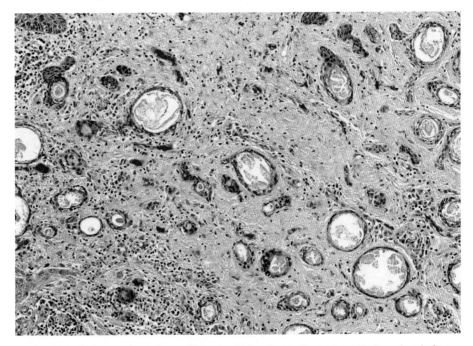

FIGURE 13.10. Syringoma is made up of bland cells forming ducts which are C-shaped and often compared to tadpoles. The duct lining is at least two layers thick. Distinction from MAC can be impossible with small superficial biopsies. Helpful distinguishing features seen in syringoma include superficial location, lack of neural invasion, and lack of atypia.

TABLE 13.2 Differential Diagnosis of MAC

Tumor	Nerve Invasion	Glandular Differentiation	Involvement of Subcutis	Cellular Morphology
MAC	Common	Present	Common	Relatively bland
DTE	Rare	Absent	Rare	Bland
BCC	Sometimes	Absent	Sometimes	Atypical
Cylindroma	Absent	Present	Absent	Bland

BCC: infiltrative basal cell carcinoma; DTE: desmoplastic trichoepithelioma; MAC: microcystic adnexal carcinoma.

approximately 20% recur and 20% metastasize to regional lymph nodes following WLE. Given the propensity for recurrence and the sometimes aggressive clinical course, MCS has been recommended.[3]

A biopsy is needed for the diagnosis. Histologically, the tumor arises from the epidermis and invades the underlying dermis (**Fig. 13.11**). Poroid tumors are composed of cells which are oval with a pink cytoplasm (**Fig. 13.12**). Small eccrine ducts (proof of eccrine origin) may be difficult to find and IHC to highlight the ducts (often CEA) may be done on the biopsy. Marked atypia and zones of necrosis and mitosis are helpful features to distinguish it from its benign counterpart, eccrine poroma (**Fig. 13.13**). The invasive front is usually quite uniform but occasionally the invasive front is highly infiltrative, perineural invasion is identified, and the tumor extends well beyond what is appreciated clinically.

IHC with CK7 is usually diffusely positive and may help with margin assessment.

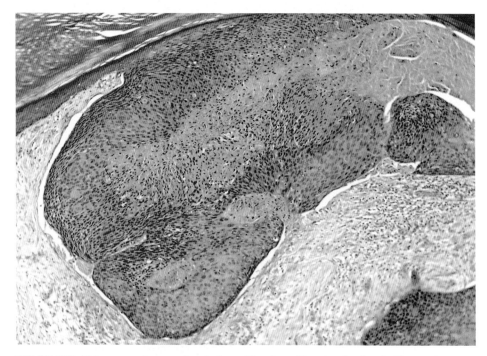

FIGURE 13.11. **This porocarcinoma arises in the epidermis and invades the dermis.** There are zones of necrosis and significant nuclear atypia.

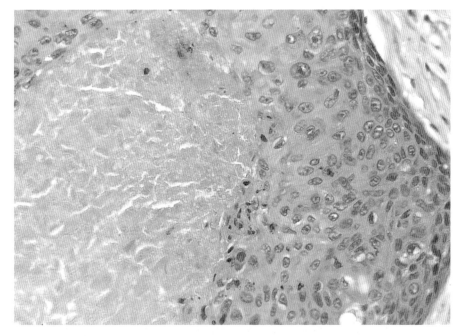

FIGURE 13.12. **High-power examination of porocarcinoma reveals that the cells have an oval nucleus and pink cytoplasm.** The malignant features here include necrosis, marked nuclear atypia, and mitoses. Well-formed ducts lined by an eosinophilic cuticle are usually seen (bottom right).

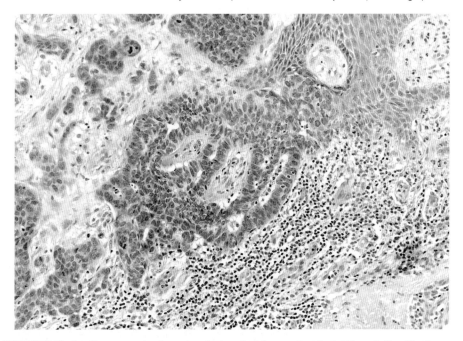

FIGURE 13.13. **Another example of porocarcinoma showing eccrine duct differentiation.** The tumor is arising from the epidermis and shows marked atypia and an infiltrative growth pattern. Due to squamous differentiation and a blue appearance, misdiagnosis as BCC or SCC is possible. In porocarcinoma, a key feature is the glandular differentiation and IHC may be needed to demonstrate this.

Hidradenocarcinoma

Hidradenocarcinoma is often a large nodular dermally based tumor arising within a benign nodular hidradenoma. Reports of hidradenoma with a fairly bland histology which have shown an aggressive clinical course can complicate the diagnosis. This has prompted some authorities to recommend the complete excision of all hidradenomas ("benign" or malignant).

A high rate of recurrence (10%-50%) has been reported with eventual metastases to lymph nodes, bones, lungs, and skin. For metastatic cases, the five-year disease-free survival is less than 30%.[4]

Histopathology usually shows a large nodular dermally based tumor which may invade the subcutaneous fat and irregularly infiltrate the surrounding dermis. The tumor cells are epithelioid, form large sheets, and have an eosinophilic cytoplasm, often with squamous areas (**Fig. 13.14**) and duct formation. Necrosis is common (**Fig. 13.15**).

Sebaceous Carcinoma

Sebaceous carcinoma arises around the eyes (ocular or periocular form), or anywhere else on the body (extraocular form). After BCC and SCC, sebaceous carcinoma is the most common eyelid malignancy where it arises from meibomian glands of tarsus, in the Zeis glands, and in the sebaceous glands of caruncle or eyebrow.

Interestingly, sebaceous carcinoma may arise sporadically or as part of Muir-Torre syndrome. This syndrome is caused by defective DNA mismatch repair genes and frequently manifests as sebaceous neoplasms as well as a range of internal malignancies. The syndrome is more common when sebaceous carcinoma arises on the trunk or limbs. Evidence of a syndromal association can be supported by IHC in which a lack of nuclear staining for

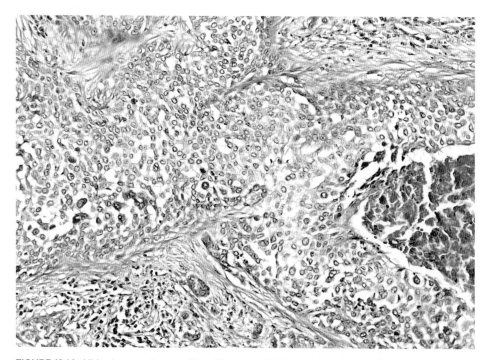

FIGURE 13.14. Hidradenocarcinoma with solid nests of highly atypical tumor cells and zones of necrosis. The cells have areas of squamous differentiation.

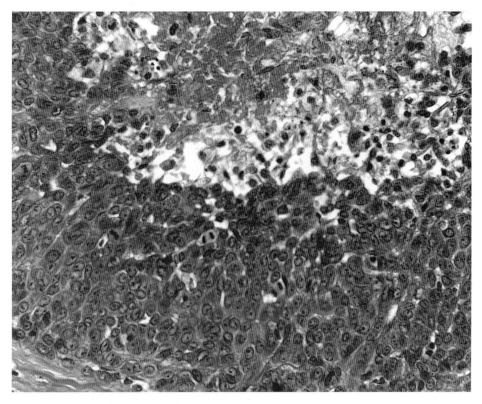

FIGURE 13.15. High-power examination of hidradenocarcinoma shows marked nuclear atypia and necrosis not seen in benign hidradenoma.

some or all of MLH1, MSH2, MSH6, and PMS2 within the sebaceous tumor is suggestive (though diagnostic) of the syndrome. Recognition of the association with internal malignancy can alert the clinical team to investigate this syndromal possibility as sebaceous carcinoma tends to precede visceral malignancies in about 60% of cases.

Recurrence is not uncommon following WLE (with or without adjuvant radiation). One study demonstrated that 9% to 36% of sebaceous carcinoma patients had local recurrence and 3% to 25% showed distant metastasis after surgery. Resection by MCS has been recommended and some studies have correlated MCS with lower recurrence and metastatic rates.[5]

Periocular cases which are advanced may require exenteration and are not generally candidates for MCS. When confined to the eyelid, wedge excisions with complete margin assessment are the usual approach. Extrocular forms can be dealt with much like other skin carcinomas.

Histopathologically, sebaceous carcinoma is composed of a mixture of markedly atypical basaloid cells invading the dermis. Key to the diagnosis is the recognition of the intermixed sebaceous cells (sebocytes). Sebocytes are large and have a large clear cytoplasm against the background of atypical basaloid cells (**Fig. 13.16**). The sebocytes are multivacuolated cells with nuclear indentation. Low-grade lesions are well-defined and composed of plenty of sebocytes while less well-differentiated tumors are more infiltrative and have fewer vacuolated sebocytes (**Fig. 13.17**).

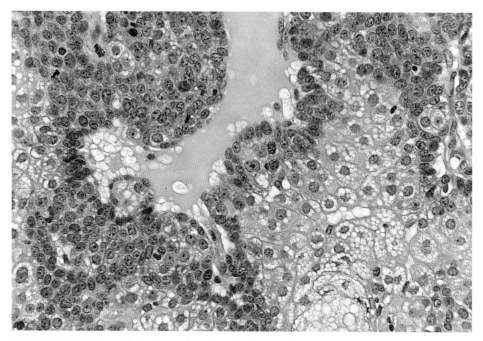

FIGURE 13.16. **Sebaceous carcinoma shows atypical basaloid cells invading the dermis with inter-mixed collections of sebaceous cells (sebocytes).** This example is a low-grade lesion with numerous sebocytes.

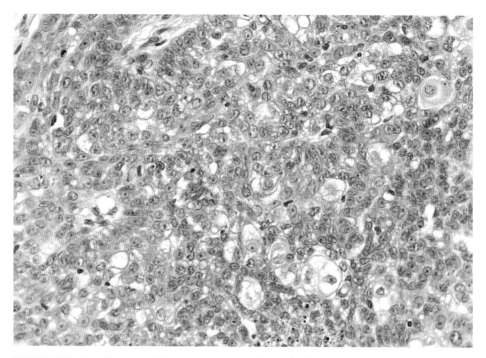

FIGURE 13.17. **Sometimes careful inspection is needed to identify sebaceous differentiation.**

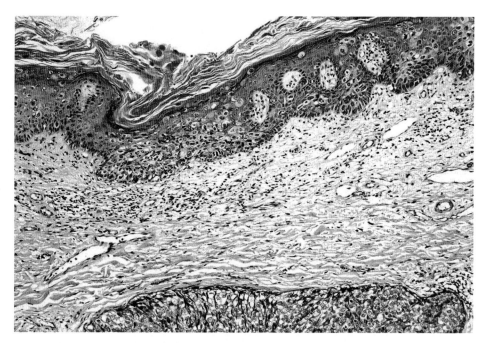

FIGURE 13.18. **Sebaceous carcinoma with invasion of the overlying mucosa is associated with a higher rate of recurrence.** This can easily be mistaken for *in situ* and invasive SCC without recognition of the sebocytes (sebocytic differentiation). (Image courtesy of Phillip McKee, Consulting Dermatopathologist and Dr. Eduardo Calonje, St John's Institute of Dermatology, London.)

Frozen section interpretation may be complicated by artifacts which cause vacuoles to appear to mimic the vacuoles of sebaceous differentiation in non-sebaceous epithelial cells. IHC can be helpful in highlighting the tumor intraoperatively. EMA, PRAME, androgen receptor, and adipophilin are the most frequently used antibodies to highlight sebaceous differentiation.

When sebaceous carcinoma involves the mucosal epithelium of the conjunctiva or the eyelid epidermis (**Fig. 13.18**), the recurrence rates have been reported to be higher than those without this feature (44% vs 30%). In cases with this feature, some have advocated doing multiple mapping biopsies before surgery as part of the planning. Adjuvant therapies (e.g., cryotherapy or topical application of mitomycin C) have also been suggested when histologic mucosal involvement is present.[6]

Eccrine Spiradenocarcinoma

Eccrine spiroadenocarcinoma usually arises within a benign eccrine spiradenoma. It typically presents as accelerated growth of a longstanding indolent lesion (**Fig. 13.19**). It is considered an aggressive tumor, with a reported recurrence rate of 57%, metastasis rate of 39%, and mortality rate of 20%. Grade of tumor has been shown to correlate with prognosis, with low-grade lesions having a much lower recurrence rate than high-grade tumors (14% vs 50%) and improved mortality (14% vs 38%).[7]

EMPSGC

This tumor almost invariably occurs in the eyelid (**Fig. 13.20**), presenting as a slow-growing papule. It is usually clinically indolent but can recur. Histopathologically, the

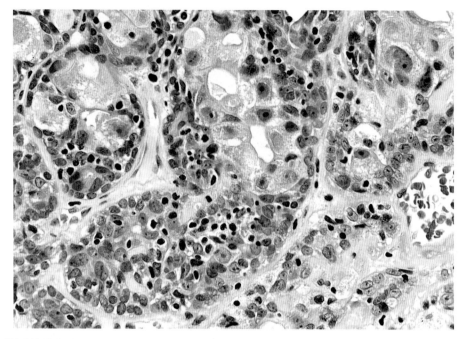

FIGURE 13.19. **Eccrine spiradenocarcinoma can show areas of benign eccrine spiradenoma (lower aspect of the photo) with sharp transitions to a malignant morphology.** The carcinoma typically shows marked nuclear pleomorphism, atypia, and mitoses. The malignant areas can be carcinomatous or sarcomatous.

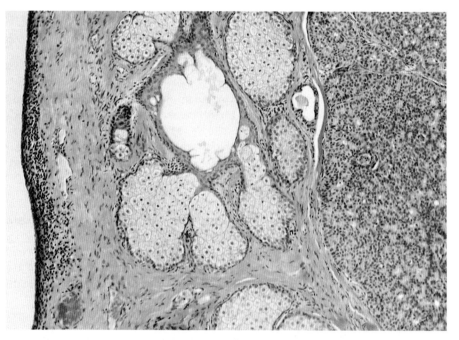

FIGURE 13.20. **A nodular tumor of EMPSGC is seen in the stroma below the sebaceous glands.** The eyelid mucosa (conjuntiva) is normal. The mucosa can be recognized by the thin epithelium without keratinization.

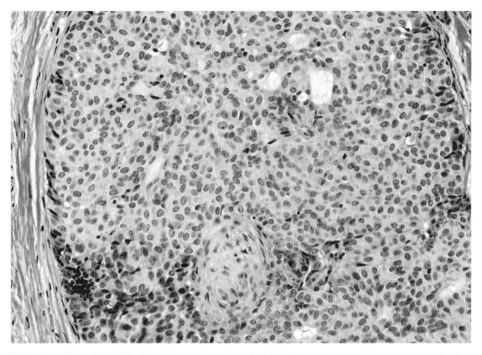

FIGURE 13.21. In EMPSGC, the cells are uniform and bland. The nuclear features are neuroendocrine with a fine, dusty chromatin. These cells show neuroendocrine differentiation with IHC for chromogranin and/or synaptophysin.

cells are uniform and bland and the nuclear features are neuroendocrine with a fine, dusty chromatin (**Fig. 13.21**). These cells show neuroendocrine differentiation with IHC for chromogranin and/or synaptophysin. Some authors have suggested that endocrine mucin-producing sweat gland carcinoma (EMPSGC) is best conceptualized as a precursor lesion, with the transition to invasive carcinoma characterized by a loss of cell polarity and mucin secretion into the tissue stroma.[8] Given the location on the eyelid and the reports of recurrence and evolution into invasive carcinoma, MCS is preferred.

Primary Mucinous Carcinoma of the Skin

Primary cutaneous mucinous carcinoma usually presents as a slow-growing mass which may be slightly translucent and blue. The eyelid is the most commonly affected site but many other sites have been described. It is associated with a high recurrence rate following WLE and the potential for aggressive local invasion. Lesions arising near the eye have a recurrence rate of 34%. Metastasis to regional lymph nodes has been reported in up to 30% of cases but metastasis to distant sites is practically unheard of. MCS offers a lower recurrence rate.[9]

The tumor is composed of clusters of epithelial cells with uniform cuboidal nuclei. The epithelial islands float in large pools of mucin (**Fig. 13.22**).

Identical tumors arise in breast and gastrointestinal sites so the exclusion of cutaneous metastasis from other sites is needed before contemplating excision. IHC has only limited utility in this distinction. A systemic evaluation is therefore mandatory before a definitive diagnosis of primary cutaneous mucinous carcinoma can be made.

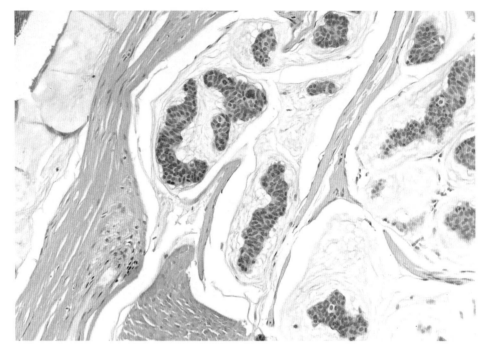

FIGURE 13.22. Mucinous carcinoma of the skin is characterized by glands and solid nests of epithelial cells floating in copious mucin.

When examining the margins, care must be taken to ensure acellular pools of mucin are not overlooked as these should be interpreted as foci of carcinoma. Subclinical spread can occasionally be extensive and result in a large defect (**Fig. 13.23**). Use of IHC (e.g., broad spectrum cytokeratin or CK7) intraoperatively can be helpful in delineating margins.[10]

Adenoid Cystic Carcinoma
Cutaneous adenoid cystic carcinoma (ACC) is less aggressive than the salivary gland counterpart and has less potential for distant metastasis. Despite this, local recurrence has been reported in 44% of cases following WLE.[11]

A range of histologic patterns can be seen including tubular, solid, and cribriform (**Fig. 13.24**). Perineural invasion has been reported in up to 76% of cases, which is a good reason to consider employing MCS to achieve clear margins while minimizing tissue defects. In cases with significant perineural invasion, a safety margin may be helpful to confirm the negative margin.

ADPA
Aggressive digital papillary adenocarcinoma (ADPA) is highly malignant and arises on the fingers and toes, usually around the nail. It frequently recurs with incomplete excision, with a recurrence rate reportedly as high as 50%. An aggressive clinical course is common, with a reported rate of metastasis ranging from 14% to 41%. ADPA has historically been treated with a radical excision, often meaning a radical amputation. MCS can be considered and may offer an alternative to amputation. Involvement of bone needs to be evaluated preoperatively.[12]

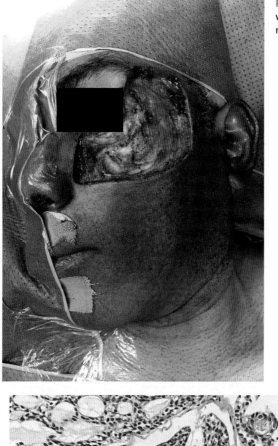

FIGURE 13.23. An extensive excision was required for complete removal of mucinous carcinoma of the eyelid.

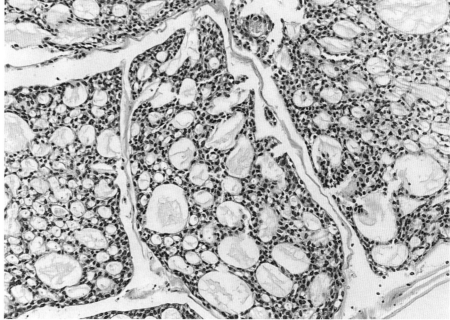

FIGURE 13.24. In adenoid cystic carcinoma, the tumor is composed of columns, nests, and islands of relatively monotonous cells arranged concentrically around pseudocystic spaces.

Despite the aggressive clinical course, the histopathology is frequently deceptively bland. Although an adenomatous form has been described, the current trend is to consider even those with a bland histopathology malignant since histopathologic grading cannot accurately predict recurrence and metastasis. The pattern of adenocarcinoma can be cystic, papillary, ductal, or solid (**Fig. 13.25**).

PHCE

Primary signet-ring cell/histiocytoid carcinoma of the eyelid (PHCE) is an adenocarcinoma of eccrine glands. It presents clinically as a smooth, bland subcutaneous nodule on the eyelid. The deceptively benign clinical diagnosis often leads to a delay in the diagnosis and significant associated morbidity. Many patients with this carcinoma initially present with features of locoregional spread such as loss of vision, neuropathic facial pain, or bony metastases.

The histopathology can also be very challenging. There is usually a subtle, diffuse dermal and subcutaneous infiltrate of single or linearly grouped epithelial cells resembling histiocytes (**Fig. 13.26**).

Recurrences are common due to incomplete tumor removal or orbital involvement. The recurrence-free period ranges from five months to eight years. Metastasis occurs in up to half of patients, especially in the regional lymph nodes. Given the high recurrence rate and diffuse infiltration, MCS offers the best chance of complete removal. The assistance of CK7 IHC to better exclude malignancy at the margins is very helpful (**Fig. 13.27**).

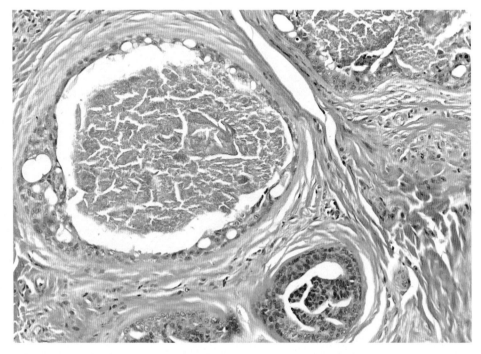

FIGURE 13.25. ADPA is an adenocarcinoma which often shows papillary projections into the lumina of glands. Extensive infiltration is usually seen.

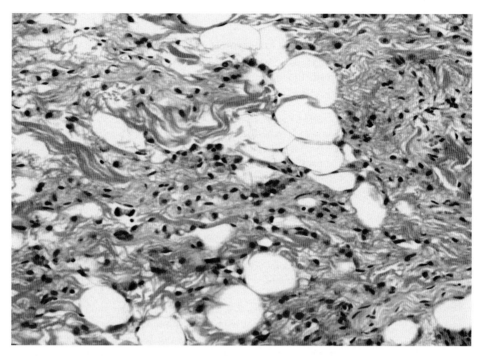

FIGURE 13.26. In PHCE, histology shows a diffuse dermal and subcutaneous infiltrate of single or linearly grouped epithelial cells exhibiting oblong or round nuclei with abundant granular cytoplasm.

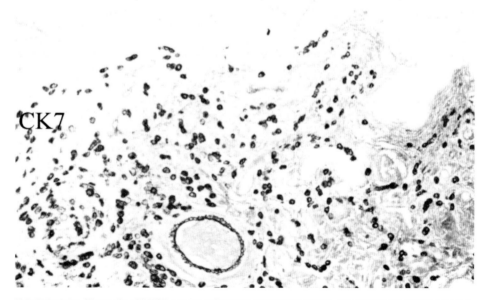

FIGURE 13.27. The cells of PHCE can be difficult to see histologically. Often IHC with CK7 is needed to highlight the extensive infiltration.

SUMMARY

Malignant adnexal tumors are a diverse group of tumors which can present some diagnostic challenges. MCS is a natural fit for these tumors, some of which spread far beyond what is perceived clinically and most of which have an improved prognosis following complete surgical excision.

References

1. Gordon S, Fischer C, Martin A, Rosman IS, Council ML. Microcystic adnexal carcinoma: a review of the literature. *Dermatol Surg.* 2017;43(8):1012-1016.
2. Diamantis SA, Marks VJ. Mohs micrographic surgery in the treatment of microcystic adnexal carcinoma. *Dermatol Clin.* 2011;29(2):185-190, viii.
3. Song SS, Wu Lee W, Hamman MS, Jiang SI. Mohs micrographic surgery for eccrine porocarcinoma: an update and review of the literature. *Dermatol Surg.* 2015;41(3):301-306.
4. Tolkachjov SN, Hocker TL, Hochwalt PC, et al. Mohs micrographic surgery for the treatment of hidradenocarcinoma: the Mayo Clinic experience from 1993 to 2013. *Dermatol Surg.* 2015;41(2):226-231.
5. Elias ML, Skula SR, Behbahani S, Lambert WC, Schwartz RA. Localized sebaceous carcinoma treatment: wide local excision versus Mohs micrographic surgery. *Dermatol Ther.* 2020;33(6):e13991.
6. Zhou C, Wu F, Chai P, et al. Mohs micrographic surgery for eyelid sebaceous carcinoma: a multicenter cohort of 360 patients. *J Am Acad Dermatol.* 2019;80(6):1608-1617.e1.
7. Beaulieu D, Fathi R, Mir A, Nijhawan RI. Spiradenocarcinoma treated with Mohs micrographic surgery. *Dermatol Surg.* 2019;45(1):152-154.
8. Scott BL, Anyanwu CO, Vandergriff T, Nijhawan RI. Endocrine mucin-producing sweat gland carcinoma treated with mohs micrographic surgery. *Dermatol Surg.* 2017;43(12):1498-1500.
9. Brownstein MH, Helwig EB. Metastatic tumors of the skin. *Cancer.* 1972;29:1298-307.
10. Marra DE, Schanbacher CF, Torres A. Mohs micrographic surgery of primary cutaneous mucinous carcinoma using IHC for margin control. *Dermatol Surg.* 2004;30(5):799-802.
11. Xu YG, Hinshaw M, Longley BJ, Ilyas H, Snow SN. Cutaneous adenoid cystic carcinoma with perineural invasion treated by Mohs micrographic surgery: a case report with literature review. *J Oncol.* 2010;2010:469049.
12. Haynes D, Thompson C, Leitenberger J, Vetto J. Mohs micrographic surgery as a digit-sparing treatment for aggressive digital papillary adenocarcinoma, dermatologic surgery. *Dermatol Surg.* 2017;43(12):1487-1489.

14

Extramammary Paget's Disease

Richard B. Johnston / Patrick Emanuel

Efficacy
Multidisciplinary Approach
Margin Processing

Histopathology
Histopathologic Mimics
Summary

Extramammary Paget's disease (EMPD) is a rare adenocarcinoma which usually presents as an enlarging erythematous plaque on anogenital skin of the elderly. It can grow slowly and is often misdiagnosed clinically as a dermatosis for years before a biopsy discovers the correct diagnosis.

EMPD infiltrates the epidermis and spreads radially as unpredictable frond-like extensions extending far beyond what is perceived clinically. Metastatic disease from adnenocarcoma of other sites (usually colorectal or prostatic) can infiltrate the epidermis and precisely mimic EMPD histopathologically. This possibility needs to be considered before surgical management is discussed.

EFFICACY

Margin control surgery (MCS) is an appealing option for these tumors due to the frequent significant subclinical spread. Review of case reports comparing those treated with conventional surgery versus MCS shows of 2.5-fold higher risk of recurrence with conventional surgery.[1] Other reports have shown a recurrence rate of 23% for MCS versus 33% for conventional surgery.[2]

MULTIDISCIPLINARY APPROACH

Cases are usually presented at a multidisciplinary meeting (MDM) to discuss the diagnosis and therapeutic options. A typical scenario would be a protracted clinical course (before the diagnosis is made) and multiple unsuccessful attempts to achieve a clear surgical margin with wide local excision (WLE). Topical or destructive therapeutic options are also often considered, especially for larger lesions. Input from dermatology as well as gynecological, urological, colorectal, and plastic/reconstructive surgeons is typically sought. The pathology is usually reviewed to confirm the diagnosis and radiology may be reviewed to further exclude the possibility of disease metastatic from an internal primary adenocarcinoma.

Radical resection often means complete vulvectomy or penectomy and without MCS these may still result in positive surgical margins. Though cases of multifocality have been described, there is mounting evidence that this is rare, if it occurs at all.[3,4]

MARGIN PROCESSING

Due to the large size of these tumors, a modified approach is often used with a complete peripheral margin assessment performed under local anesthetic (with the central tumor left intact) followed by the excision of the central tumor under general anesthetic. Sometimes the tumor is so ill-defined that it is not clear *where* the excision of the first level should be performed. In these cases, scouting biopsies may be used to help roughly determine the extent of disease. Biopsies that sample the maximum amount of epidermis (e.g., broad-shave biopsies) are preferred. Reflectance confocal microscopy may also help in the delineation.[5] The radial margin is removed as a thin strip, mapped, and embedded *en face* for examination of the entire margin. This is sometimes called the "spaghetti" technique[6] (**Fig. 14.1**).

The margin assessment may be processed intraoperatively with frozen sections or in paraffin if the patient is to return for surgery the next day. When the tumor approaches or invades cutaneous-mucosal interfaces such as the urethra, vagina, or anus, a complete circumferential margin of the mucosa is also needed to confirm full clearance.

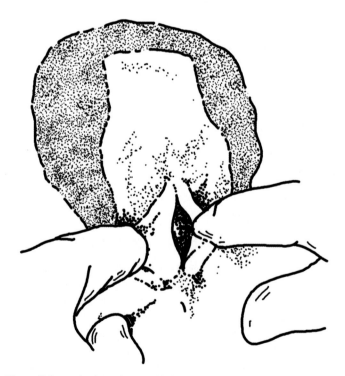

FIGURE 14.1. The radial margins have been entirely removed in strips and processed *en face* for complete radial margin assessment (sometimes called the spaghetti technique). Inner mucosal margins lateral to the urethra and vulva also need to be examined to ensure complete removal before excision of the central tumor.

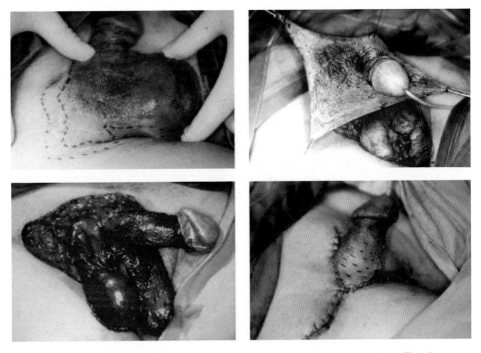

FIGURE 14.2. In this case of EMPD of the scrotum, the visible tumor was marked out. The disease was far more extensive than anticipated. Tracking the margins histologically resulted in this patient requiring a complete scrotectomy and skin grafting with the testis placed in an inguinal pouch.

Following complete radial (and mucosal) clearance, the main tumor mass is excised with a generous deep margin (preferably to fascia) to ensure clearance of any follicular or glandular extension of the carcinoma. This central specimen should be sent in formalin for paraffin sections. Often the reconstruction is complex and relies on the expertise of multiple specialists including plastic and reconstructive, urological, and gynecological surgeons (**Fig. 14.2**).

HISTOPATHOLOGY

In EMPD, tumor cells infiltrate the epidermis. The tumor cells are large with a clear or eosinophilic cytoplasm, have large pleomorphic nuclei, and show marked atypia (**Figs. 14.3** and **14.4**). In rare cases, an underlying adnexal carcinoma (e.g., apocrine adenocarcinoma) may be present in the dermis.

Tumor cells contain abundant mucin which can be identified by staining with Alcian blue and periodic acid-Schiff. Immunohistochemically, Paget cells stain for EMA, cytokeratins, and variable positivity for CEA. Lesions confined to the epidermis are usually CK7 positive and CK20 negative (**Fig. 14.5**).

HISTOPATHOLOGIC MIMICS

As mentioned earlier, the key to the diagnosis is the exclusion of metastasis (**Table 14.1**) from another site and other histopathologic mimics (**Table 14.2**). Distinction usually requires immunohistochemistry (IHC).

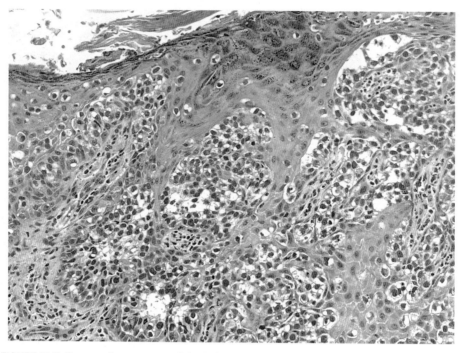

FIGURE 14.3. **Tumor cells are scattered throughout the epidermis.** The tumor cells are large and often have a clear or eosinophilic cytoplasm as well as large pleomorphic nuclei. Sometimes the tumor cells form glands.

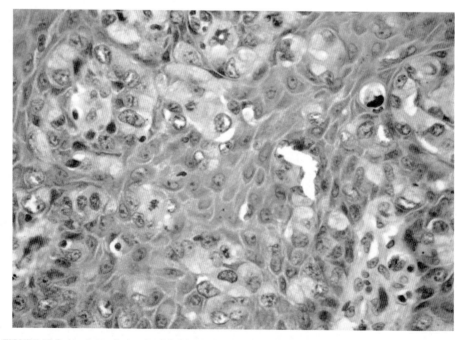

FIGURE 14.4. **In cases where glandular formation is not evident, the tumor can mimic melanoma or SCC.** In such cases, confirmation with IHC is needed.

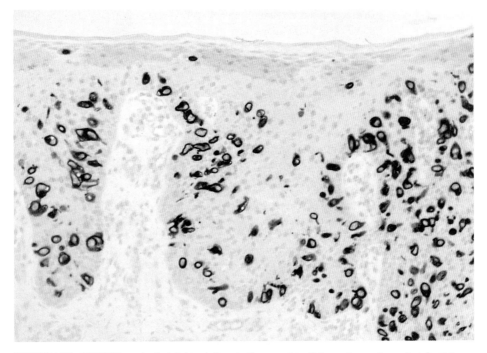

FIGURE 14.5. CK7 IHC can be helpful to delineate the margins. This can be performed on frozen section material (as seen here) or in paraffin sections.

TABLE 14.1 Basic Immunohistochemical Panel to Exclude Metastasis

	CK7	CK20	CDX2	PSA
EMPD	+	−	−	−
Colonrectal cancer	−	+	+	−
Prostatic cancer	−	−	−	+

TABLE 14.2 Basic Immunohistochemical Panel to Exclude Other Primary Tumors

	CK7	CK20	Her2	EMA	P63	Melan-A
EMPD	+	−	−	+	−	−
SCC	−/+	−	−	−	+	−
Melanoma	−	−	−	−	−	+

Melanoma *in situ:* In contrast to EMPD, melanoma is negative for cytokeratins, EMA, and CEA. Sox-10 and Melan-A are usually negative in EMPD and positive in melanoma.

Bowen disease: P63 is positive in Bowen disease, differentiating it from EMPD. It should be noted that cytokeratin 7 may be positive in both EMPD and Bowen disease.

Mammary Paget's Disease: This condition is morphologically identical but arises from an underlying carcinoma of the breast. IHC is generally not helpful in providing precise distinction but extramammary Paget's disease often lacks the Her-2/neu expression seen in some cases of the mammary disease.

EMPD always needs to be considered when these other diagnoses are made on genital skin. Liberal use of IHC to confirm the diagnosis is recommended.

SUMMARY

EMPD is a rare adenocarcinoma occurring on genital skin of the elderly. By the time it is diagnosed, it typically involves a large area, has ill-defined margins, and may involve genital mucosal surfaces. MCS plays a central role in achieving clear surgical margins. A multidisciplinary approach is recommended, particularly in complex cases.

References

1. Long B, Schmitt AR, Weaver AL. A matter of margins: surgical and pathologic risk factors for recurrence in extramammary Paget's disease. *Gynecol Oncol.* 2017;147(2):358-363.
2. Yao H, Xie M, Fu S, et al. Survival analysis of patients with invasive extramammary Paget disease: implications of anatomic sites. *BMC Cancer.* 2018;18(1):403.
3. Zhao Y, Gong X, Li N, Zhu Q, Yu D, Jin X. Primary extramammary Paget's disease: a clinico-pathological study of 28 cases. *Int J Clin Exp Pathol.* 2019;12(9):3426-3432.
4. Long B, Schmitt AR, Weaver AL. A matter of margins: surgical and pathologic risk factors for recurrence in extramammary Paget's disease. *Gynecol Oncol.* 2017;147(2):358-363.
5. Terrier JE, Tiffet O, Raynaud N, Cinotti E. In vivo reflectance confocal microscopy combined with the "spaghetti" technique: a new procedure for defining surgical margins of genital Paget disease. *Dermatol Surg.* 2015;41(7):862-864.
6. Gaudy-Marqueste C, Perchenet AS, Taséi AM. The "spaghetti technique": an alternative to Mohs surgery or staged surgery for problematic lentiginous melanoma (lentigo maligna and acral lentiginous melanoma). *J Am Acad Dermatol.* 2011;64(1):113-118.

SECTION IV
Case Reports and Discussions

15

Case 1. Basic Basal Cell Carcinoma

Patrick Emanuel / Mark Izzard

Details of the process of margin control surgery (MCS) may seem daunting to a skin surgeon contemplating its introduction to their practice. This simple basal cell carcinoma (BCC) illustrates how straightforward the process can be. Doctors who refer out MCS cases may wish to explain the process to patients by showing them a case like this one.

An 82-year-old man was referred for MCS with a lesion on the cheek. It had grown slowly over months and had recently started to crust and bleed (**Fig. 15.1**). Clinically, it was thought to be a classic nodular BCC.

Following the usual preoperative procedures (including discussion of the procedure and consents), the lesion was demarcated with a pen (**Fig. 15.2**). Dermatoscopy helped to delineate the margins radially.

Local anesthetic was injected (**Fig. 15.3**).

Curettage was performed (**Fig. 15.4**). The patient did not have a preoperative biopsy, so the curettage biopsy was immediately processed as a frozen section to confirm the diagnosis of BCC. The tumor extended further than expected with the curettage and a new margin was demarcated with a pen and a notch made for orientation (**Fig. 15.5**).

The first level was excised (**Fig. 15.6**). The bevel angle was around 45°.

The specimen was orientated by creating a single notch. As this was a small uncomplicated lesion, a single notch was sufficient. The specimen was carefully laid out on a gauze with the notch facing a blue spot drawn on a gauze. The patient label was attached to the gauze for identification (**Fig. 15.7**).

Ink was placed on either side of the notch on the specimen (**Fig. 15.7**).

The defect was dressed (**Fig. 15.8**) and the patient returned to the waiting room while the slides were processed. Anesthetic (as needed) was administered.

The specimen was embedded in frozen section medium using a slide to facilitate a perfectly flat margin (see Chap. 6). Horizontal sections were cut in the cryostat and stained with routine hematoxylin and eosin. These slides showed BCC present at a radial margin, on the green side of the notch (**Figs. 15.9** and **15.10**). This was drawn on the corresponding map.

The second level was drawn on the patient with a pen to encompass the positive margin as indicated on the map. This was excised, orientated with a notch, drawn on a map, and processed with frozen section examination as done with the first level to allow complete examination of the new radial margin.

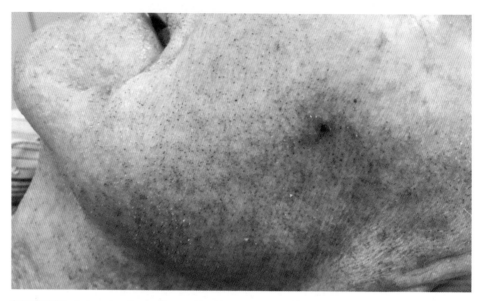

FIGURE 15.1. **A slow-growing lesion on the cheek raises suspicions of BCC.** Dermatoscopy helps illustrate arborizing vessels, telangiectasia, and focal ulceration.

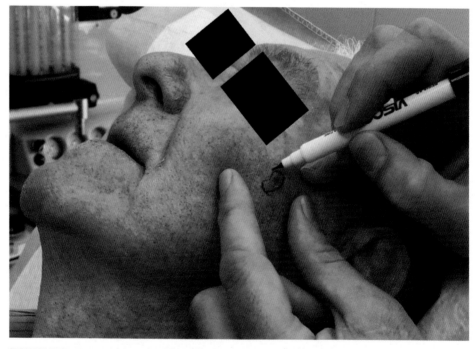

FIGURE 15.2. **The tumor was demarcated with a pen.** Magnifying glasses, the zoom function on a smartphone, or a dermatoscope can aid in demarcation.

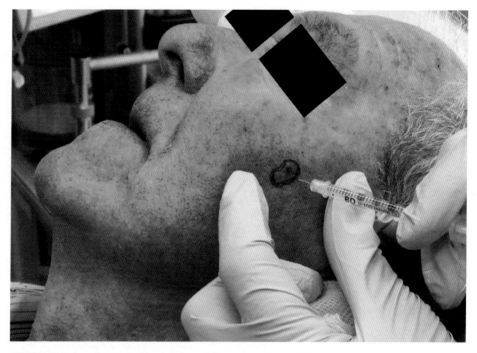

FIGURE 15.3. **Local anesthetic was injected.** Extending the local infiltration to well beyond the tumor markings is advised since the next step, curettage, may extend well beyond the initial margin.

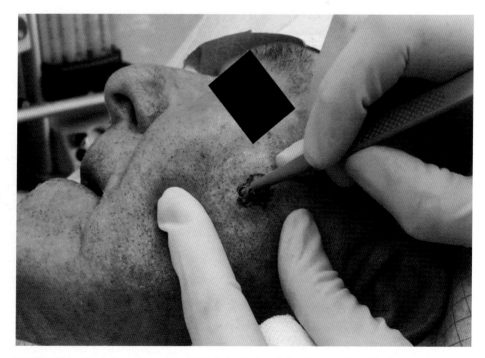

FIGURE 15.4. **The tumor was curetted.** This helps further define the margins of the tumor.

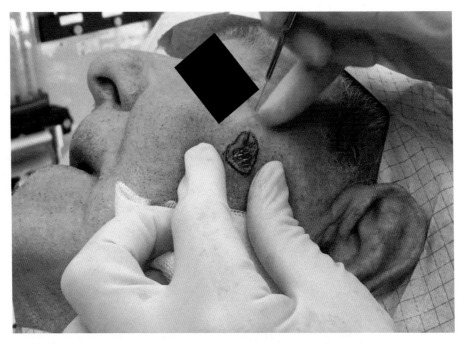

FIGURE 15.5. **The delimitation of the margin was redrawn as the tumor extended slightly further with the curette than initially anticipated.** 1-2 mm of intact epithelium is generally needed around the defect for the excision. A notch was cut for orientation.

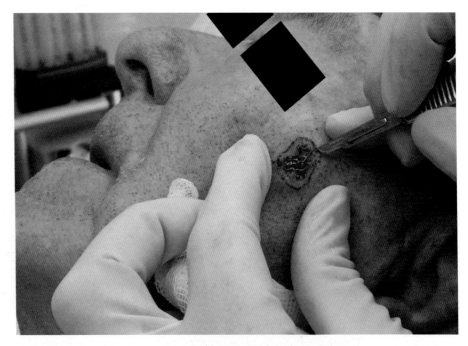

FIGURE 15.6. **Following curettage and marking, the first level was excised.** The bevel angle of around 45° allows for easier embedding of the specimen.

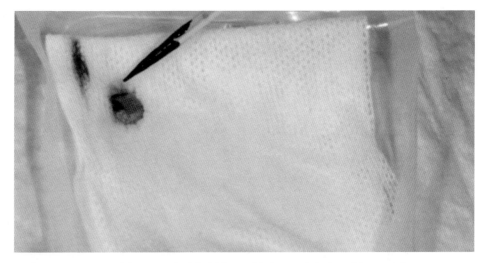

FIGURE 15.7. **The specimen was carefully laid out with the notch facing a blue spot drawn on gauze.** The patient label was attached to the gauze for identification. There are many techniques described for orientation including sutures, double notches, and so on. Whichever method is chosen, one which is simple, reproducible, and allows precise mapping will eliminate error. This specimen was inked with blue and green inks on either side of the notch.

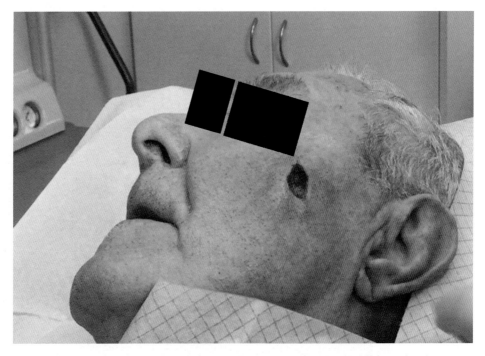

FIGURE 15.8. **The defect was dressed with a hemostatic substance (such as Kaltostat) and a pressure dressing applied.** Further oral or local anesthetic may be administered while the patient waits for slide processing.

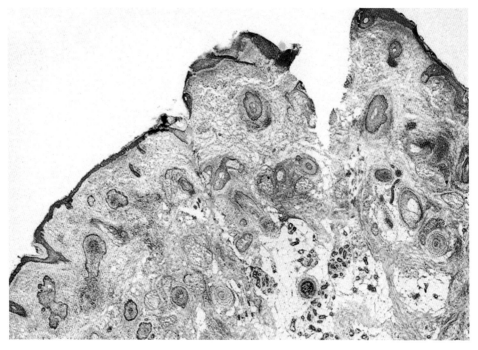

FIGURE 15.9. **The first level was examined with a frozen section.** The notch and the colors blue and green are clearly visible.

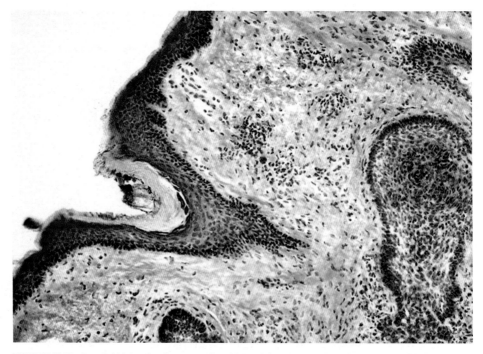

FIGURE 15.10. Basaloid islands of tumor cells with peripheral palisading diagnostic of BCC are clearly seen at the radial margin, close to the notch on the green side of the specimen.

Histologic assessment revealed no residual tumor. The wound was closed with a simple linear closure.

The entire procedure in this case lasted approximately two hours, during which the patient relaxed in the waiting room for most of the time.

Some important points are worth emphasizing.

This patient arrived without a histopathologic diagnosis. It was incumbent on the team to submit the curetted specimen for an immediate frozen section to confirm the clinical suspicion before beginning surgery. In some practice settings, an external pathology report is needed for reimbursement. In that scenario, the frozen biopsy tissue can be submitted in formalin to an outside laboratory following the frozen section diagnosis.

The curettage of the tumor discovered that the tumor was larger than initially appreciated with the clinical exam. This illustrates how important curettage can be for delimiting the margin prior to excision. Often the curettage will remain within the original drawn line. However, if the size of the lesion is underestimated or overestimated, a new margin will need to be drawn. A good 1 to 2 mm of peripheral intact epithelium around the curettage defect is ideal for the excision.

The bevel angle of 45° was important to process the specimen as it allows for easier flattening of the margin for the *en face* horizontal sectioning technique (see Chap. 6).

The first level was positive radially. If this patient had had a WLE with standard processing, the excision would have been larger and resulted in a larger facial scar. Perhaps more importantly, with routine paraffin processing, the margin may have been assessed as being positive (and the patient would have been subjected to a second operation for re-excision) *or* the routine paraffin sectioning may have missed the positive margin (as only a small fraction of the margin was examined) and the tumor would have been far more likely to recur.

It is worth being conscious of the possible causes for error in a basic case like this so they can be avoided:

- *Incorrect orientation.* This is minimized with the surgeon cutting an orientating notch, orientating it on the piece of gauze, and drawing the details immediately on the corresponding map.
- *Not enough overlap.* The second level needs to include the entire area of positivity in the first level. Errors arise when the second level does not extend sufficiently to encompass this positive area, in which case the second level could spuriously be considered negative histopathologically. Less experienced surgeons may be inclined to excise generous second levels to avoid this.
- *Flipping of the second level.* Significant care must be taken with the second level to ensure the true new surgical margin is embedded flat and examined. If the other side is examined by mistake (the side closest to the tumor rather than the new surgical margin), this will likely cause the second level to be incorrectly read as positive.

16

Case 2. Large Facial Lentigo Maligna

Patrick Emanuel / Mark Izzard

There are few things more frustrating for a skin surgeon than a pathology report—from a wide excision that required a complex reconstruction—detailing multiple positive surgical margins.

A 68-year-old woman with a history of multiple skin cancers presented with a large asymmetric pigmented lesion on the cheek. It had very irregular borders, a range of colors from light brown to black, and had apparently slowly increased in size over a few years (**Figs. 16.1** and **16.2**).

A deep incisional biopsy was performed. Histologic examination confirmed melanoma *in situ*, lentigo maligna (LM) type, extending to the radial margins. No dermal invasion was identified.

A routine wide local excision (WLE) was performed with a 5-mm margin around the clinically visible tumor (**Fig. 16.3**). Routine histopathology showed LM in this excision, extending to within 2 mm of the radial margin in the sections examined. Somewhat surprisingly, a further re-excision revealed small foci of residual LM extending to within 1.25 mm of a radial margin.

Finally, a further excision with 5-mm margins was performed and this was found to be negative for malignancy (**Fig. 16.4**). The workflow of this case is outlined in **Table 16.1**.

The scenario illustrated in this case is not too uncommon when dealing with LM of the face. This patient was subjected to four separate surgical procedures. Each was performed on different days over several weeks while the pathology was being processed and examined, and the next surgical procedure was booked only once the pathology report was received in the surgeon's office.

LM is well known to extend histopathologically much further than is appreciated clinically or dermatoscopically. To ensure that the illustrated LM had been completely excised with the first excision attempt, an excision with up to 15-mm margins (around the visible lesion) would have been needed. The majority of LM does not need an excision of anywhere near this size.

In one of the excisions, the LM was thought histopathologically to have been completely excised with narrow measured pathological margins (2 mm) yet the subsequent excision revealed further disease. This illustrates the inherent inaccuracy of bread loaf margin assessment of WLE specimens, as only a small fraction of the entire margin is examined.

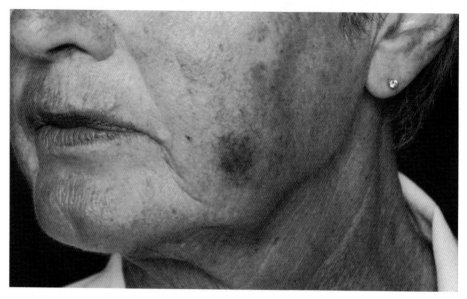

FIGURE 16.1. **A highly atypical pigmented lesion on the cheek.**

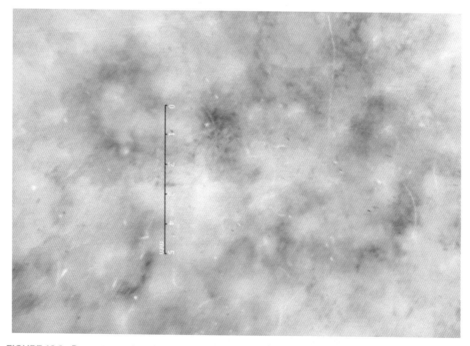

FIGURE 16.2. **Dermatoscopic examination confirmed a highly atypical lesion.** There is a pseudo network, asymmetric pigmented follicular openings, and white scar-like areas.

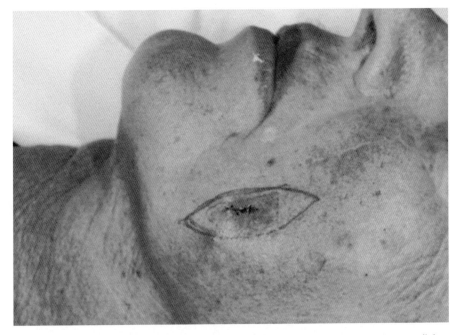

FIGURE 16.3. After the diagnosis had been confirmed with the biopsy, a 5-mm-minimum radial margin was drawn around the identified tumor.

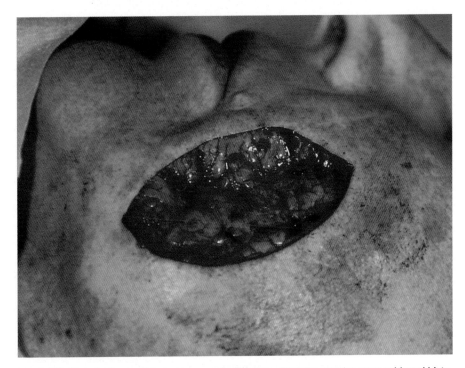

FIGURE 16.4. Two further excisions were required before adequate margins were achieved histopathologically, resulting in a large defect.

TABLE 16.1 Workflow of Illustrated Case

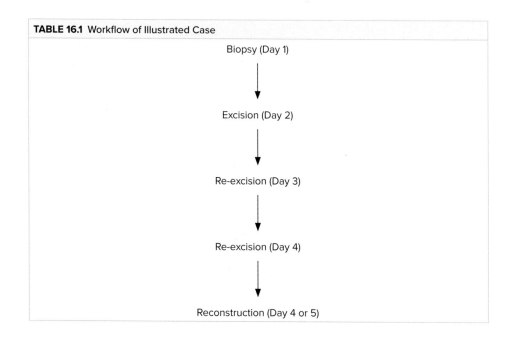

Biopsy (Day 1)

↓

Excision (Day 2)

↓

Re-excision (Day 3)

↓

Re-excision (Day 4)

↓

Reconstruction (Day 4 or 5)

Key considerations as to how this tumor could have been managed differently and with margin control surgery (MCS) include the following:

(i) **Biopsy.** A deep incisional biopsy as performed in the illustrated case is appropriate. However, for flat pigmented lesions on the head and neck, a shave biopsy which permits maximum histopathologic examination of the epidermis offers an excellent alternative. Broad shave biopsies have the additional benefit of providing an excellent cosmetic result in the case where the lesion is benign (e.g., macular seborrheic keratosis, lentigo simplex). The shave biopsy should also sample the superficial reticular dermis so that superficial invasion can be identified. If deeper invasion of a thick melanoma is suspected clinically, a deeper incisional biopsy is needed and superficial shave biopsies should be avoided. Immunohistochemistry to assess subtle early dermal invasion can be performed on shave biopsies.

(ii) **Debulk.** Though clinical assessment gives some idea as to the extent of LM in many cases, sometimes this assessment is impossible. With MCS, instead of a 5-mm margin being drawn around visible tumor, a narrow 1-mm margin would be drawn and excised. This would be sent as a debulk specimen to the laboratory for paraffin examination to exclude subtle invasion.

(iii) **Excision.** The management of the illustrated case failed because the chosen excision margin was basically *guesswork*. In contrast, with MCS, a narrow additional margin around the debulk defect would be excised. This margin would be entirely examined intraoperatively with *en face* frozen sections. The margins would be positive, and these would be drawn on a corresponding map. Positive margins would be re-excised immediately and again examined immediately. This process would be repeated until the margin was clear of tumor.

(iv) **Pathologic examination.** Using telepathology, the margins could have been examined intraoperatively with a dermatopathologist. Various techniques to facilitate

TABLE 16.2 Alternative Workflow Using MCS

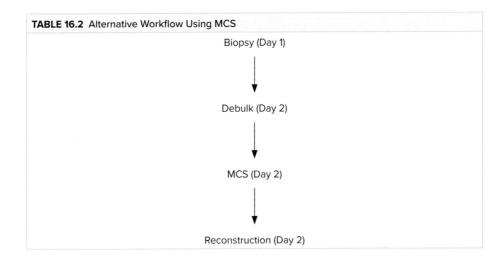

Biopsy (Day 1)

↓

Debulk (Day 2)

↓

MCS (Day 2)

↓

Reconstruction (Day 2)

telepathology are available. A smartphone with microscope adapter offers a cheap, convenient, and accurate method of intraoperative consultation.[1]

(v) **Reconstruction.** Once the tumor was clear with intraoperative frozen sections, an additional safety margin (1-2 mm) might have been removed for paraffin examination. This would give further reassurance that the LM has been completely excised and the surgeon may elect to wait for this confirmation before reconstruction. However, reconstruction is usually performed on the same day and before the results of this paraffin examination. Cases which are histopathologically challenging may benefit from immunohistochemistry to ensure the final margins are negative.

The procedure could have occurred with two visits (the first for the biopsy and the second for excision and reconstruction) instead of the four outlined in the illustrated case. The cost would have been markedly lower, the entire process would likely have caused the patient less anxiety, and the resulting defect would likely have been smaller (**Table 16.2**).

There are a variety of methods which can be used to perform MCS for LM (see Chap. 11). The precise method is less relevant provided that the entire margin is examined, and that the expectations of the surgeon and pathologist are communicated and well understood.

Reference

1. Emanuel PO, Patel R, Zwi J, Cheng D, Izzard M. Utility of teledermatopathology for intraoperative margin assessment of melanoma in situ, lentigo maligna type: a 6 year community practice experience. *Eur J Surg Oncol.* 2021;47(5):1140-1144.

17

Case 3. Microcystic Adnexal Carcinoma

Patrick Emanuel / Mark Izzard

It's a misconception that skin cancers are invariably "prosaic" basal cell carcinoma (BCC), SCC, or malignant melanoma. Skin cancers are fascinatingly varied and complex. Microcystic adnexal carcinoma (MAC) is a good example of an underappreciated skin cancer which can be misdiagnosed, inadequately excised, and highly destructive.

An 84-year-old woman presented for margin control surgery (MCS) with a tumor of the cheek which had been previously biopsied and diagnosed as a BCC. The slides were reviewed prior to the surgery. The pathologist noted that areas of the biopsy showed a highly infiltrative growth pattern, areas of ductal differentiation, and infiltration of small nerves. These findings were interpreted as more in line with a MAC rather than a BCC (**Fig. 17.1**).

MCS was performed. The first excision was a central scalpel debulk which was sent to an outside laboratory in formalin for paraffin processing (**Fig. 17.2**). This facilitated a comprehensive histopathologic examination and confirmed the diagnosis of MAC. The first level was excised with approximately 2-mm clinical margins around the central debulk defect. The first-level histologic sections showed extensive tumor involving the entire radial margin (**Fig. 17.3**). The deep margin was negative for malignancy. The case was discussed with a remote dermatopathologist using a telepathology system utilizing an adapter and smartphone with a teleconference application.

Three further levels were needed to achieve negative margins. At this point, almost the entire cosmetic subunit had been removed, so the remainder of that subunit was then demarcated and removed. This specimen served as a safety margin which was embedded in paraffin for margin assessment (**Figs. 17.4** and **17.5**). The defect was left open until the safety margin was confirmed to be negative for malignancy. Due to the size of the defect and its location, quite a meticulous reconstruction was needed (**Fig. 17.6**).

This case highlights several important points.

It is ideal to review the histopathology of biopsy specimens preoperatively. Sometimes superficial biopsies can be extremely difficult to interpret correctly. This is particularly true for sclerosing facial tumors where distinguishing between BCC, trichoepithelioma, and MAC can be difficult (see Chap. 8). In the current case, the correction to the diagnosis was made preoperatively, so the appropriate planning could take place. Sometimes the correct diagnosis only comes to light intraoperatively when frozen section examination

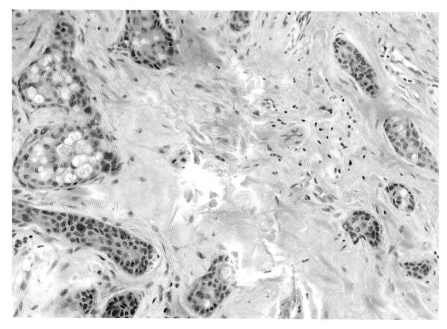

FIGURE 17.1. Review of the pathology shows an infiltrative basaloid tumor with ductal differentiation consistent with MAC.

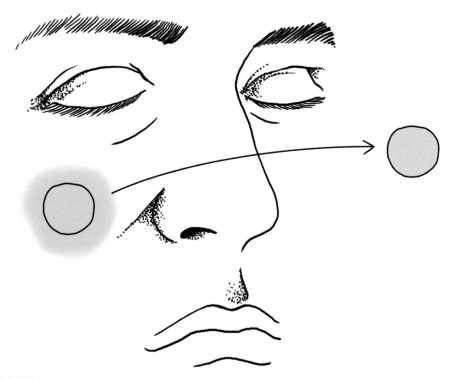

FIGURE 17.2. A central debulk was excised and sent in formalin to an outside laboratory for comprehensive study and diagnosis.

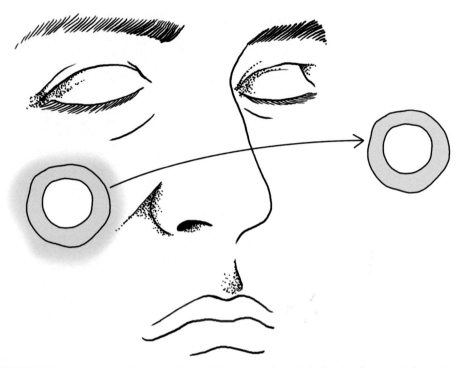

FIGURE 17.3. Intraoperative frozen sections of the margin showed the first level was entirely positive radially. The deep margin was clear.

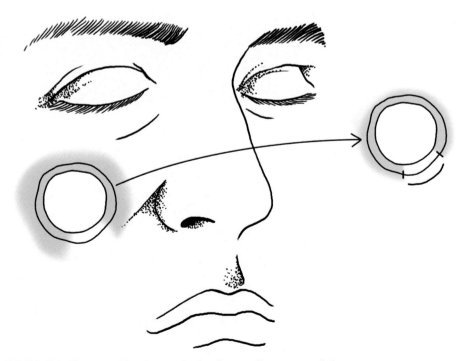

FIGURE 17.4. The second level was only clear in a small segment radially.

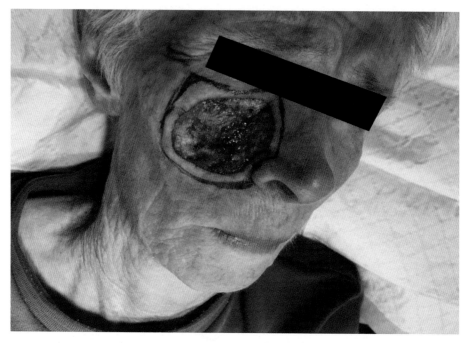

FIGURE 17.5. Following four levels, the resulting defect was just short of encompassing the entire cosmetic subunit. The remainder of the subunit was excised and served as a safety margin. This was negative for malignancy.

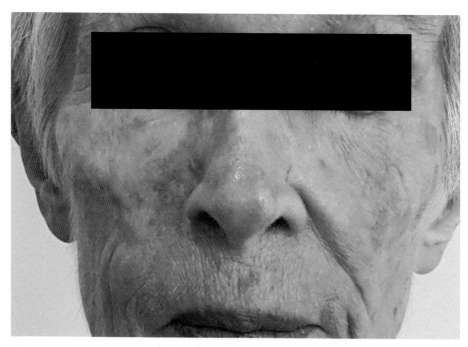

FIGURE 17.6. The defect was repaired with a full-thickness skin graft resulting in a good cosmetic result.

discovers diagnostic features not evident or overlooked in the preoperative biopsy. Because of this, a re-evaluation of the surgical approach may need to be considered in real time. This re-evaluated approach may include schedule issues (a longer procedure is expected), and consideration given to more extensive surgery (such as a nerve dissection and/or a final safety margin excision).

The case highlights the utility of MCS in assessing the extent of the tumor. A regular excision would have eventuated in positive margins and quite likely multiple surgical efforts would have been needed to clear the tumor. Additionally, if the margins had been evaluated with a regular bread loaf histopathology assessment, a spuriously negative margin may have been assessed. MAC is notorious for its high recurrence rate and much of the reason for this appears to be inadequate margin assessment/inadequate surgical excision in the initial surgical management. Recurrence of MAC on facial skin can be devastating, often consisting of extensive invasion of deep tissues and nerves.

The use of a telepathology system allowed real-time evaluation of the morphology with a dermatopathologist. The popularity of remote pathology has dramatically increased due to technological innovations and more recently due to necessity caused by the COVID-19 pandemic. Real-time evaluation where both the surgeon and the dermatopathologist view slides together is comparable to using a multiheaded microscope. As the slides are viewed, pertinent clinical and pathologic aspects of the case can be discussed and the margins can be interpreted and mapped together.

Finally, it is helpful for the surgeon to consider the final surgical defect in the context of the planned reconstruction. If the reconstruction intends to replace an entire cosmetic subunit, it makes sense to use the excised subunit as a safety margin as was done in the illustrated case.

18

Case 4. Dermatofibrosarcoma Protuberans of the Scalp

Patrick Emanuel / Mark Izzard

While tumor recurrence and mortality rates are easy things to measure, cosmetic outcomes are relatively subjective and receive less attention in the literature. For large malignancies arising on cosmetically or functionally sensitive skin, *margin control surgery* (MCS) offers the dual benefit of a complete excision and the sparing of normal tissue. MCS minimizes the chance of an incomplete excision and maximizes the chance of a good cosmetic outcome.

A 33-year-old man presented with what was thought to be a 2.5-cm benign cyst on the scalp. It had been present for several years and the patient thought it had slowly been growing. His family doctor aimed to completely excise the "cyst" by performing a small elliptical excision.

Histopathology showed a spindle cell tumor consistent with dermatofibrosarcoma protuberans (DFSP) (**Figs. 18.1** and **18.2**). Immunohistochemistry (IHC) with CD34 (**Fig. 18.3**) and molecular studies confirmed this diagnosis.

The patient was referred for a specialist evaluation and he sought multiple specialist opinions.

An MRI revealed that the lesion measured approximately 4 cm in maximum dimension and that it approached—but did not invade—bone. CT-PET scan revealed no evidence of metastasis.

At one tertiary surgical oncology center, he was offered a wide local excision (WLE) with 2-cm clinical margins. This plan would have involved direct reconstruction and routine (likely bread loaf) pathologic examination of the margins. Postoperative radiotherapy was also recommended, with permanent alopecia over a large area of the scalp being an expected consequence.

The patient was referred to our service and discussed at the multidisciplinary meeting (MDM) which included members from head and neck surgery, radiology, pathology, and oncology, as well as nursing staff. After discussion, the recommendation was for MCS using frozen section examination of the entire margin intraoperatively. This recommendation is in line with the current National Comprehensive Cancer Network® (NCCN) guidelines which recommend MCS for all cases of DFSP where possible.

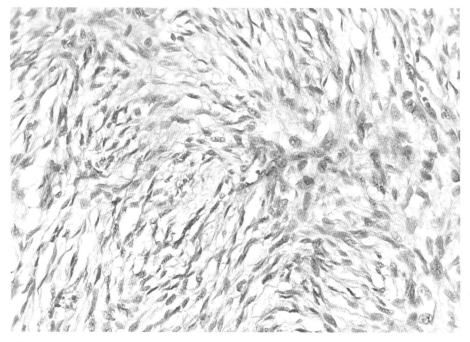

FIGURE 18.1. Histopathology showed a spindle cell tumor composed of slender tumor cells embedded uniformly in the collagen stroma without significant mitotic activity. In some areas, there was a high cellularity and irregular, short, intersecting bands of tumor cells forming a storiform and cartwheel pattern.

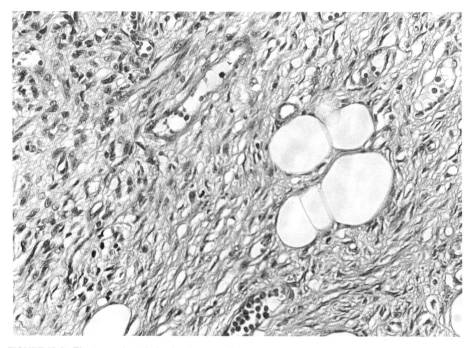

FIGURE 18.2. The tumor invaded subcutaneous fat.

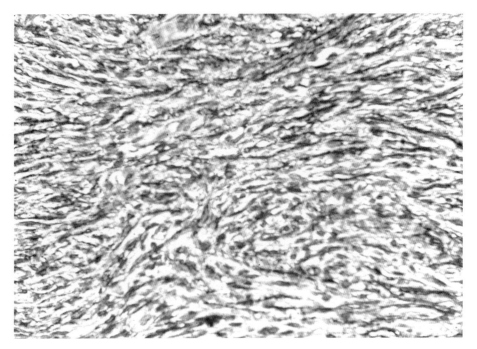

FIGURE 18.3. IHC with CD34 was positive, as is seen in almost all cases of DFSP. Melanoma markers (S100, Sox10, not shown) were negative. The diagnosis was confirmed with molecular studies.

MCS was performed using the *en face* 3D technique outlined in Chap. 6. The first level was more like a large mapping biopsy as the extent of the tumor was difficult to discern clinically. Not surprisingly, there was extensive involvement of the margins of the first level and these were mapped on the corresponding orientation map. Four subsequent levels guided by the positive margins found intraoperatively were excised to achieve complete removal of the tumor. The resulting defect measured up to 14 cm in its largest dimension (**Fig. 18.4**).

Due to the large size of the tumor and the subtle nature of the histopathology, an additional safety margin was excised (**Fig. 18.5**) and processed in paraffin for *en face* histopathologic examination and IHC (CD34) of the entire radial surgical margin. Because the MRI had demonstrated proximity to bone, the bone at the deep margin was curetted and this specimen was sent separately as the deep margin and processed urgently.

The open defect was dressed and the patient was discharged. The negative margin was confirmed both with the paraffin sections of the radial safety margin (including the CD34 IHC) and the bone curettings of the deep margin. A reconstruction was performed and resulted in an excellent cosmetic outcome (**Figs. 18.6** and **18.7**).

The case was discussed again at the MDM where it was decided that radiotherapy was not needed at that time. Four years have elapsed and close clinical and radiologic follow-up shows no evidence of recurrence. Most recurrences occur within three years of the primary excision, so this is reassuring.

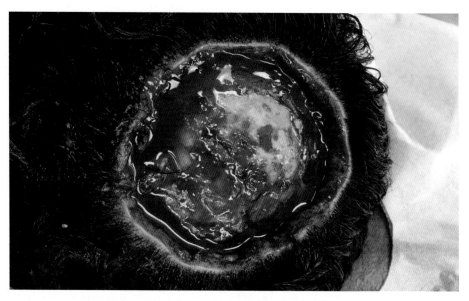

FIGURE 18.4. **Multiple excised levels were positive for DFSP with frozen section examination.** Following frozen section clearance of the tumor, the defect was quite large.

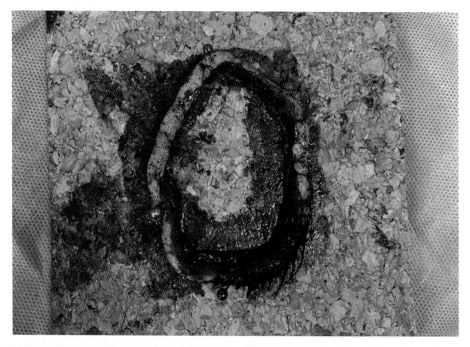

FIGURE 18.5. **An additional safety margin of the peripheral margin was removed as a ring and orientated.** This was embedded in paraffin *en face* to allow examination of the entire margin and, as expected, showed no evidence of residual disease. IHC with CD34 was also performed to confirm the negative radial margins.

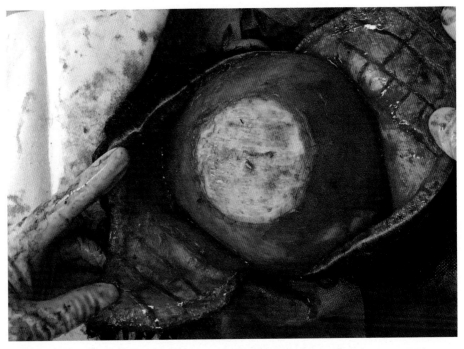

FIGURE 18.6. Following confirmation of the negative margins, the defect was reconstructed.

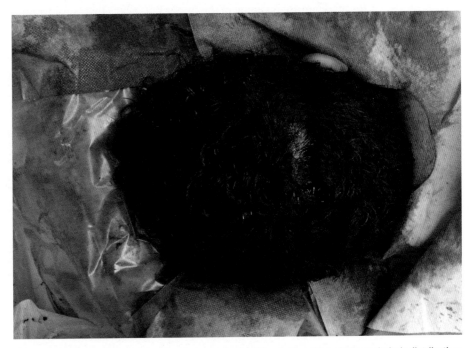

FIGURE 18.7. The cosmetic outcome was excellent, without disruption of the scalp hair distribution.

This case is instructive for a few reasons.

DFSP has a protean clinical presentation. It can be mistaken for various disorders including a desmoid scar, cyst, burn, dermatofibroma, or an acrochordon. The fact that this case was initially mistaken for a cyst illustrates the importance of the histopathologic examination of all skin biopsies or excisions for diagnosis, regardless of the clinical suspicion.

Accurate histopathologic diagnosis is key to stratifying risk and managing sarcomas. The utilization of ancillary tests provides further diagnostic confidence. In the case of DFSP, the characteristic genetic alteration is present in 80% to 90% of cases and can be identified with FISH genetic testing which is widely available and was used in the presented case. A positive result not only confirms the diagnosis but also implies a continuous activation of the PDGF-β signaling pathway which can be targeted with therapy. This targeted therapy (e.g., imatinib) is usually reserved for inoperable, neoadjuvant, or metastatic settings.

Given the difficulty in assessing DFSP on frozen sections, a final safety margin which is processed in paraffin is often helpful. As the reconstruction is often performed on a later day, the safety margin usually does not delay the process much if at all. In paraffin sections, the morphology is easier to interpret and IHC for CD34 can be performed to provide further reassurance that the final margins are clear.

It is worth noting that in this case the tumor extended well beyond the anticipated excision margin which had been planned with a WLE. In addition, as far as we were aware, the WLE had not planned to use methods to assess the entire margin, so it is possible that the margins would have been erroneously determined to be negative. In cases like this, it is helpful to treat the first level as more of a mapping biopsy with the anticipation that the margins will be positive in areas rather than doing a radical excision upfront. This allows for more precise mapping of the tumor but means that consideration needs to be given to the surgeon's schedule for the day since the procedure may last for some time as multiple levels are likely to be needed.

Many centers opt to do MCS with rapid paraffin section processing rather than using intraoperative frozen sections. In the case illustrated here, five separate surgical procedures may have been needed for complete excision. Faced with this scenario, the surgeon is often tempted to opt for a radical wide surgical margin with the first level, risking cosmetic and functional compromise.

Finally, the planned radiotherapy was not considered necessary following the complete surgical excision. This not only ensures the cosmetic advantage of the patient retaining his scalp hair but also avoids the side effects of radiotherapy.

Three quite distinct surgical strategies are outlined in **Table 18.1** to emphasize the advantages of the strategy used in the presented case.

TABLE 18.1 Treatment Option Summary

TREATMENT OPTION 1: WLE WITH ROUTINE PROCESSING

Excision with 2-cm margin without complete margin assessment and reconstruction (one operation). This risks falsely interpreting the margins as negative if the entire margin is not examined. Most likely, the margins would be determined to be positive, necessitating further excisions and reconstructions. WLE is no longer considered a surgical option for DFSP in the NCCN unless complete margin assessment is not available.

↓

Postoperative radiotherapy. Permanent alopecia and possible radiotherapy complications.

TREATMENT OPTION 2: MCS WITH RAPID PARAFFIN PROCESSING RATHER THAN INTRAOPERATIVE FROZEN SECTIONS

Excision with rapid processing of entire surgical margin in paraffin. The margins would be positive and continue to be positive with five subsequent excision attempts resulting in at least five operations

↓

Reconstruction following confirmation of negative margins. The outcome would likely have been the same as for the presented case, but the multiple operations would have been hugely costly and inconvenient.

TREATMENT OPTION 3: MCS WITH INTRAOPERATIVE FROZEN SECTIONS AND FINAL SAFETY MARGIN IN PARAFFIN (AS DONE IN THE PRESENTED CASE)

Margins evaluated intraoperative with frozen section examination. A long procedure was needed but complete excision was achieved in one session. A final safety margin is sent for rapid paraffin examination to confirm negative margins.

↓

Reconstruction following confirmation of negative paraffin safety margin. The physicians can have a high level of confidence that the tumor has been completely excised. Radiotherapy was not applied.

19

Case 5. Pleomorphic Dermal Sarcoma of the Scalp

Patrick Emanuel / Mark Izzard / Edgar Jesus Salas Moscoso

Confusing nomenclature can put patients at risk. Atypical fibroxanthoma (AFX) is a low-grade malignancy of the dermis associated with minimal risk. Pleomorphic dermal sarcoma (PDS) likewise involves the dermis but also invades subcutaneous tissue and carries a slightly higher risk of recurrence and metastasis. Undifferentiated Sarcoma (also commonly called malignant fibrous histiocytoma) arises in deeper soft tissues and has a dismal prognosis. The cells of all these tumors look identical microscopically. Confusing these terms can result in unnecessary radical surgery, radiotherapy, and even chemotherapy in some cases. Psychological sequelae from incorrectly assigning a highly malignant diagnosis can also be devastating.

A 62-year-old man with a history of multiple previous skin cancers presented with an enlarging ulcerated tumor on the scalp measuring 3 cm in its greatest clinical dimension. A superficial biopsy had been performed and the histopathology revealed a tumor composed of highly atypical pleomorphic tumor cells with sarcomatoid features. No *in situ* disease was evident in the epidermis. Immunohistochemistry (IHC) was performed on the biopsy and revealed no evidence of squamous differentiation (CK5/6, p63), melanocytic differentiation (Sox-10, Melan-A), vascular differentiation (CD31), or smooth muscle differentiation (desmin). A diagnosis of AFX was made.

This patient was referred for margin control surgery (MCS), but the initial slides were not available for review. A biopsy was performed on the day of surgery and examined fresh with frozen sections (**Fig. 19.1**). The pathology matched that described in the biopsy report, i.e., the tumor was undifferentiated and pleomorphic. The tumor was overt histopathologically so not challenging to see in the frozen section slides and therefore a good candidate for intraoperative margin assessment.

MCS proceeded and evaluation of the entire margin was performed with the *en face* 3D technique (see Chap. 6). The radial margins were clear, but the tumor was noted to extend deep into subcutaneous adipose tissue (**Fig. 19.2**). This is a feature not typically seen in AFX and generally suggests a diagnosis of PDS.

Given the unusual deep involvement, the tissue excised in the first level and frozen for margin assessment was placed in formalin and sent to the pathology laboratory for paraffin processing as a debulk specimen.

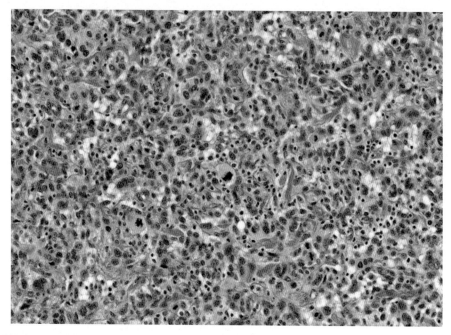

FIGURE 19.1. **A biopsy on the day of surgery showed a highly atypical pleomorphic tumor without clear differentiation consistent with the referred diagnosis of AFX.** Intraoperative biopsy is helpful as it offers a glimpse of the expected morphology in the margin evaluation.

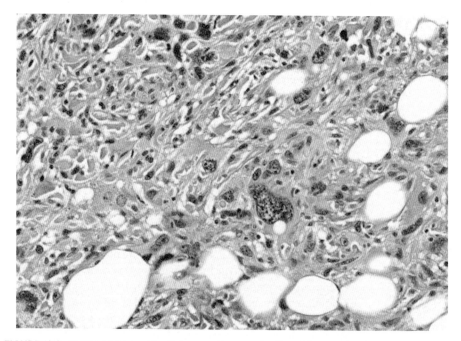

FIGURE 19.2. **During intraoperative frozen section examination of the margins, it was noted that the tumor extended deeply into subcutaneous tissues.** This is not a feature typically seen in AFX and suggests a diagnosis of PDS.

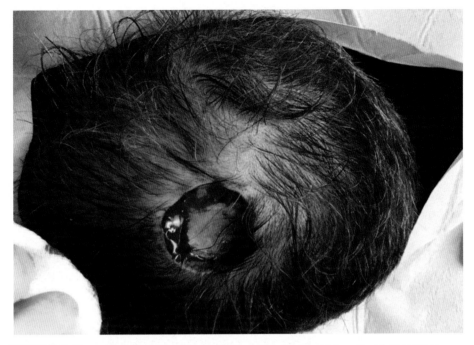

FIGURE 19.3. **The entire tumor was cleared with the second level which excised further tissue radially and deep tissue (down to pericranial tissues).** The defect was closed in the same surgical session. The case was discussed at an MDM and no additional therapy (e.g., radiotherapy) was recommended.

The entire tumor was cleared with the second level which included an excision down to pericranial tissue (**Fig. 19.3**). The defect was closed on the day of surgery.

Following the surgery, the patient was discussed at a multidisciplinary meeting (MDM). The pathology report from the paraffin examination of the debulk was concordant with the intraoperative findings, i.e., there was an invasion deep into the subcutaneous fat consistent with a PDS. No invasion of vessels or nerves was noted. This specimen had been resubjected to IHC which again failed to reveal evidence of differentiation toward a melanocytic, epithelial, vascular, or smooth muscle lineage. The main question of the meeting was whether radiotherapy to the site was required. After presentation of the case and discussion of the current literature, radiotherapy was not recommended. The patient is now six years post-operative and there is no indication of metastasis or recurrence. The workflow is outlined in **Table 19.1**.

This case highlights that an understanding of the pathology is critical in treating these tumors surgically. AFX and PDS show the same morphology with histopathologic examination of superficial biopsies. But the latter is usually larger (>2 cm) and displays additional aggressive histologic features usually not evident in biopsy specimens, namely, extensive subcutaneous invasion, necrosis, and invasion of vessels and nerves. When any of these features are seen intraoperatively, the surgeon needs to be aware that distinguishing AFX from PDS is clinically relevant. The prognosis of AFX is excellent and, following complete excision, a good outcome is almost universally achieved. PDS has a higher quoted rate of local recurrence and metastatic disease. Additionally, care needs to be taken to ensure that

TABLE 19.1 Workflow of Current Case

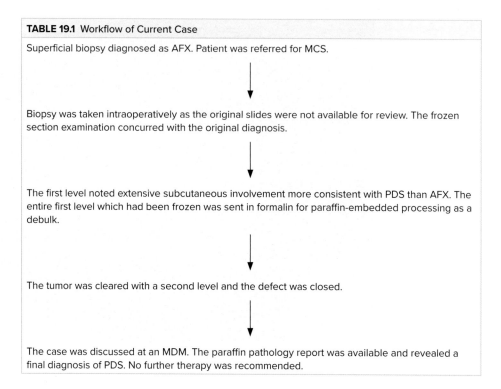

Superficial biopsy diagnosed as AFX. Patient was referred for MCS.

Biopsy was taken intraoperatively as the original slides were not available for review. The frozen section examination concurred with the original diagnosis.

The first level noted extensive subcutaneous involvement more consistent with PDS than AFX. The entire first level which had been frozen was sent in formalin for paraffin-embedded processing as a debulk.

The tumor was cleared with a second level and the defect was closed.

The case was discussed at an MDM. The paraffin pathology report was available and revealed a final diagnosis of PDS. No further therapy was recommended.

the tumor is examined thoroughly with paraffin examination and IHC stains to rule out an unusual melanoma, carcinoma, or other sarcoma. For this reason, sending a debulk of the tumor for paraffin assessment is usually prudent. Presenting these cases at an MDM is almost always worthwhile to review the clinical features, pathology, and possible use of adjuvant therapies such as radiotherapy.

Index

NOTE: italics indicates a figure; boldface indicates a table.

A

AAD. *See* American Academy of Dermatology (AAD)
acantholytic cSCC *117, 118*
ACC. *See* adenoid cystic carcinoma (ACC)
Actinic keratosis (AK) 18, *19*
adenoid cystic carcinoma (ACC) 190, *191*
adenosquamous carcinoma *117*
adnexal tumors *176–177, 178–180*
    ACC 190, *191*
    ADPA 190–192, *192*
    biopsy 175–176
    debulk 176, *176*
    differential diagnosis for MAC 180, **182**
    eccrine spiroadenocarcinoma 187, *188*
    EMPSGC 188–189, *188–189*
    general considerations 175–176
    hidradenocarcinoma 184, *184–185*
    MAC 176, *177, 178–180*
    mapping 176
    PBHCE 192, *193*
    porocarcinoma 180–182
    primary cutaneous mucinous carcinoma 189–190, *190, 191*
    safety margins 176
    sebaceous carcinoma 184–187, *186–187*
    types of 176–193
    workflow for **176**
ADPA. *See* aggressive digital papillary adenocarcinoma (ADPA)
AE1/AE3 86, **86**
AEIOU 165
AFX. *See* atypical fibroxanthoma (AFX)
aggressive digital papillary adenocarcinoma (ADPA) 190–192, *192*
AJCC. *See* American Joint Committee on Cancer (AJCC)
American Academy of Dermatology (AAD) 18, 32
American Joint Committee on Cancer (AJCC) 12, 33

anatomy, operating to 36
angiosarcoma 159–161, *160–161*
anticoagulation 21
appropriate use criteria (AUC) 18, **20**
arborizing vessels 92
Area H 18
Area L 18, **20**
Area M 18
atypia **141**, 142, **142**
atypical fibroxanthoma (AFX) 147, 148–152, *148*, **152**, 159, 231, *232*
AUC. *See* appropriate use criteria (AUC)

B

barriers to MCS 29–30
basal cell carcinoma (BCC) xvi, 18, *204*
    basaloid epithelial tumor 95, *95*
    biopsy 94–95
    case study 203–209, *204–208*
    classification of **96**
    clinical photographs *25*
    evidence 92
    examination 92–94, *93*
    fibroepithelioma of Pinkus type *99*
    high-risk **31**, 97, 100
    histopathology 95–100, *95–101*, 102
    immunohistochemistry 86
    indication guidelines for MCS 30
    infiltrative 92, *94*, 97
    low-risk 96–97
    and MCC 171
    micronodular 97, *98*
    misdiagnosis *103–108*
    nodular 92, 96–97
    overview 91
    recurrent 102
    risk stratification 95–102

basal cell carcinoma (BCC) (*Cont.*):
    sarcomatoid *99*
    subtypes 97, 100
    superficial 92, *93*
basaloid epithelial tumor 95, *95*
basaloid follicular hamartoma *104*
basaloid islands *208*
basosquamous carcinoma *100*
BCC. *See* basal cell carcinoma (BCC)
bevels 45, *45*
biases 11
biopsy
    of adnexal tumors 175–176
    of BCC 94–95
    control 130
    of cSCC 113
    of lentigo maligna 214
    of melanoma 128–129
    site identification 21
    types of 36–38, *37–38*
black swan events 111
Bowen disease 199
bread loaf technique 54–59, *55–57, 58*, **59**
Brigham and Women's Hospital (BWH) 33–34, **34**
British Association of Dermatologists 32, *33*
BWH. *See* Brigham and Women's Hospital (BWH)

C
cancer staging protocols 32–34, **34**
carcinoma IHC **86**
cartilage 71
case studies
    BCC 203–209, *204–208*
    dermatofibrosarcoma protuberans 223–229, *224–225, 226–227*
    large facial lentigo maligna 211–215, *212–213*
    MAC 217–221, *217–220*
    pleomorphic dermal sarcoma 231–234
CCPDMA. *See* continuous complete peripheral and deep margin assessment (CCDPMA)
CD10 152
CD20 *124*
CD34 86–87, 153, *155, 225*
chronic lymphocytic leukemia 123, *123*
CK5/6 **86**
CLIA. *See* Clinical Laboratory Improvement Amendments (CLIA)
clinical controls 84
Clinical Laboratory Improvement Amendments (CLIA) 14
clinical margin
    assessment xv

definition xvii
clinical marking 38–39, *39*
clinicopathologic correlation 11
coagulation 21
cognitive biases 11
COL1A1-PDGFB fusion. *See* fluorescent in situ hybridization (FISH)
complete circumferential peripheral and deep margin assessment (CCPDMA) 66
confidence interval xvi
continuous complete peripheral and deep margin assessment (CCDPMA)
    criteria for xi
    NCCN criteria **31**
control biopsy 130
cost-effectiveness, of MMS 25
COVID-19 14
cryostat cutting *63*
cSCC. *See* cutaneous squamous cell carcinoma (cSCC)
curettage 36, *37*, 205
cutaneous angiosarcoma 159–161, *160–161*
cutaneous leiomyosarcoma 156–159, *157–159*
cutaneous lymphadenoma *108*
cutaneous sarcomas
    AFX 148–152, *148–151*
    angiosarcoma 159–161, *160–161*
    DFSP 152–156
    general considerations 147–148
    leiomyosarcoma 156–159, *157–159*
    mimickers 161
    PDS 148–152, *149, 150*, 231–234
    workflow for **152**
cutaneous squamous cell carcinoma (cSCC) *113–114*
    acantholytic *117, 118*
    adenosquamous carcinoma *117*
    biopsy 113
    burden 111–112
    clinical presentation 112, *112*
    clinical risk factors **114**
    debulk 121
    desmoplastic *118*
    evidence 112
    histology risk factors 117
    histopathology 113, *114–119*
    infiltrative *122*
    keratinization 114, *115*
    and leukemia 123, *123*
    lymphatic invasion *119*
    and lymphoproliferative disease 121–123
    metasasis versus primary 123
    multidisciplinary approach 121
    perineural invasion 119, *120, 122*

pitfalls 121–124
risk stratification 114–119
safety margins 124
and sialometaplasia 124
squamous differentiation *116*
and syringometaplasia 124, *125*
variants 117
cylindroma *103*
cytokeratin 86, 102, *125*

D

debulk
  of adnexal tumors 176, *176*
  considerations in 70
  of lentigo maligna 214, *218*
  in melanoma 129, **130**, **131**
  overview 38
  in specimen preparation 65
  in sSCC 121
demarcation *204*, *213*
depth of excision 42, *43*
depth of invasion 100
dermatofibrosarcoma protuberans (DFSP) 32,
        153–156
  case study 223–229
  CD34 *225*
  cosmetic outcome *227*
  histopathology *224*, 228
  overview 152–156
  reconstruction *227*
  slide preparation and immunohistochemistry
        86–87
  spindle cell tumor *224*
  treatment option summary **229**
  workflow for **157**
desmoplastic cSCC *118*
desmoplastic trichilemmoma *106*
desmoplastic trichoepithelioma *105*, 180, *180*
DFSP. *See* dermatofibrosarcoma protuberans (DFSP)
direct method of IHC 80

E

eccrine porocarcinoma 180–182, *182–183*
eccrine spiroadenocarcinoma 187, *188*
efficacy 21, 92
EMPD. *See* extramammary Paget's disease (EMPD)
EMPSGC. *See* endocrine mucin-producing sweat gland
        carcinoma (EMPSGC)
endocrine mucin-producing sweat gland carcinoma
        (EMPSGC) 188–189, *188–189*
en face sectioning 5, 6, *24*, 59–66, *59–65*, *66*
  3D technique 66–69, *67*, *68*, **69**, *69*

excision 214
excision margin xvii
extramammary Paget's disease (EMPD)
  histopathology 197, *198–199*
  margin processing 196–197, *196–197*
  MCS efficacy 195
  mimickers 197–200, **199**
  multidisciplinary approach 195–196
  overview 195

F

fat 71, *74*
fibroepithelioma of Pinkus type *99*
fibrosarcomatous transformation 156, *157*
FISH. *See* fluorescent in situ hybridization (FISH)
fixation 78
"fixed-tissue" method 5
fluorescent in situ hybridization (FISH) *153*
follicular basaloid proliferation *108*
folliculocentric basaloid proliferation 102
"fresh-tissue" method 5
frozen section pathology 3–4

G

guesswork 35–36

H

HE. *See* hemotoxylin and eosin (HE)
hemotoxylin and eosin (HE) 77–78, **78**
hidradenocarcinoma 184, *184–185*
histologic controls 84
histology
  cSCC **117**
  high-risk BCC 97, 100
  low-risk BCC 96–97
histopathology
  of BCC 95, *95–101*, 102
  of cSCC 113, 114–119
  of cutaneous leiomyosarcoma 156
  of DFSP 153
  of EMPD 197, *198–199*
  of lentigo maligna 137–144, **138–144**
  of MAC 178
  of MCC 168–171
  pitfalls 102
  of sebaceous carcinoma 185
history
  early attempts at intraoperative diagnoses 3
  frozen section pathology 3–4
  intraoperative margin assessment 4–5
  Mohs micrographic surgery 4–6
hybrid technique *133*

I

immunohistochemistry (IHC) 6, 78, 80, *83*, 102, **131**
  clinical and histologic controls 84
  for cutaneous angiosarcoma 159
  for cutaneous sarcomas 147, **150**
  DFSP 86–87
  for EMPD mimics 197–200, **199**
  for lentigo maligna 142, **143**
  for MCC **169**, *172*
  for melanoma 85–86, **85**
  method 80, 84, **84**
  nonmelanoma skin cancers 86, **86**, *87*
  other tumors 87
  problems 84
indication guidelines for MCS 30–34
indirect method of IHC 80, *83*, **84**
indurated erythematous plaque *112*
infiltrating follicular structures *139*
infiltrative basaloid tumor *218*
infiltrative BCC 92, *94*, 97, *98*, 180, *181*
infiltrative pattern 47–51
infiltrative sSCC *122*
informed consent 21
inking 42, 53–54, *54*
intent 41
intraoperative margin assessment 4–5
intraoperative MCS outside of the MMS setting 9–16
  general workflow **10**
  multidisciplinary meetings 11–13
invasive desmoplastic melanoma **131**

K

keloid scar 161, *162*
keratinization **114**, *115*

L

layers 39
leiomyosarcoma 156–159, *157–159*
lentigo maligna *212–213*
  case study 211–215
  workflow **214**, **215**
lentigo maligna (LM) *130*
  histopathology 137–144, **138–144**
  overview 128
lentigo maligna melanoma (LMM) 128
leukemia 123, *123*
levels *40*
  bevels 45, *45*
  definition 39
  first 40–45, *48*
  second and subsequent 45–46, *48*, 209
  standard ring first level 42, *42*

lichenoid infiltrates **140**
linguine technique 132
LM. *See* lentigo maligna (LM)
LMM. *See* lentigo maligna melanoma (LMM)
lymphatic invasion *119*
lymphoproliferative disease 121–123

M

MAC. *See* microcystic adnexal carcinoma (MAC)
malignant adnexal tumors. *See* adnexal tumors
malignant fibrous histiocytoma 231
mammary Paget's disease 199–200
mapped excision 59, 137
mapping 39–40, *40*, 176
margin control surgery (MCS)
  barriers to 29–30
  compared with WLE 92
  for DFSP 153
  efficacy of 92, 195
  as equivalent procedures xi–xii
  indication guidelines for 30–34
margins xv
  clinical margin assessment xv
  guidelines comparison **xvi**
  mathematics xvi–xvii
  pattern/behavior 47, *49*
  safety 50, *50*, 71, *72–73*
  size of xvi
MCC. *See* Merkel cell carcinoma (MCC)
MCS. *See* margin control surgery (MCS)
MDMs. *See* multidisciplinary meetings (MDMs)
Melan-A 85, 142, **143**
melanocytic density 86
melanoma. *See also* melanoma in situ (MIS)
  and biopsy 128–129
  and bread loaf technique 59
  control biopsy 130
  first level 130
  histopathology 137–144
  immunohistochemistry 85–86, **85**
  indication guidelines for MCS 32
  invasive 134, *135–137*
  mapped excision 137
  specimen processing techniques 132–137, *133–137*
  suitability for MCS 127–128
melanoma in situ (MIS) 18. *See also* melanoma
  and debulk 129, **130**, **131**
  as EMPD mimic 199
  indication guidelines for MCS 32
  lentigo maligna 128
  MCS efficacy 128
  MCS suitability 127–128, **128**, *129*

Merkel cell carcinoma (MCC) xv, 18, *166*
  and BCC 171
  differential diagnosis **169**, 171, *172–173*
  examination 165–166
  histopathology 168–171, *169–170*
  IHC for **169**
  indication guidelines for MCS 32
  less-advanced tumors 166
  more-advanced tumors 166–168
  overview 165
  and SCC *170*
  surgical management strategies 166–168, *167–168*
microcystic adnexal carcinoma (MAC) 176, *177, 178–180*, **182**
  case study 217–221, *217–220*
Micrographic Dermatologic Surgery 22
micronodular BCC 97, *98*
MMS. *See* Mohs micrographic surgery (MMS)
modified MMS 132
Mohs micrographic surgery (MMS)
  advantages of 19–21
  appropriateness in Area L **20**
  clinical photographs *25*
  compared with multidisciplinary approach 10–11, **11**
  compared with WLE 19, 20–21
  cost-effectiveness 25
  definition 17–18
  efficacy 19–21
  history of 4–6
  indications for 18
  overview 132
  practical issues 21
  reconstruction 22
  recurrence rates **20**
  specimen preparation 22, *23, 24*
  surgical procedure 21–22
  tissue preservation 21
  training surgeons and technicians 22–24
  UK criteria **33**
Mohs technique of specimen preparation 59–66, *59–65*, **66**, *66*
Muir-Torre syndrome 184
multidisciplinary approach 9–16
  compared with MMS 10–11, **11**
  for cutaneous sarcomas 147
  for EMPD 195–196
  for lentigo maligna 144
  MDMs 11–13
  slow Mohs 15, **16**
  in sSCC 121
  telepathology 13–14

multidisciplinary meetings (MDMs) 11–13
  compared with MMS **11**
  criteria for **12**
  utility of **12**
multifocal growth 47–51
Munich technique 69, *69*, **70**

N
National Comprehensive Cancer Network (NCCCN) xi, xvii, 12
  case study 223
  indication guidelines for MCS 30–32, **31**
NCCN. *See* National Comprehensive Cancer Network (NCCCN)
nodular BCC 92, 96–97
nodular fasciitis 161, *162*, 165
nonmelanoma skin cancers **33**, 86, *87*
nontargeted resections 45, *46*
notches, orientation 42, *43, 44*

O
operating to anatomy 36
operating to pathology 36
orientation 209
orientation notches 42, *43, 44*
overlap 209

P
p40 86, **86**, 124
p63 86, **86**, 102, 124
paraffin IHC 80
pathological margin xvii
pathologic examination 214–215
pathology. *See also* telepathology
  frozen section. *See* frozen section pathology
  history of 3
  operating to 36
  and specimen preparation 53
patient locator 42
pattern/behavior at margin 47
PBHCE. *See* primary signet-ring cell/histiocytoid carcinoma of the eyelid (PHCE)
PDEMA 66
PDS. *See* pleomorphic dermal sarcoma (PDS)
perimeter technique 70
perineural invasion (PNI) 100, *101*, 113, 119, *120*, *122*
peripheral and deep *en face* margin assessment (PDEMA) 66
peripheral sectioning of wedge excisions 70, **71**, *71*
physiognomy 77

pleomorphic dermal sarcoma (PDS) 148–152, *149, 150*
  atypical fibroxanthoma *232*
  case study 231–234, *232–233*
  workflow for **152, 234**
PNI. *See* perineural invasion (PNI)
porocarcinoma 180–182, *182–183*
PRAME. *See* PReferentially expressed Antigen in
    Melanoma (PRAME)
PReferentially expressed Antigen in Melanoma (PRAME)
    86
primary cutaneous mucinous carcinoma 189–190, *190,*
    191
primary signet-ring cell/histiocytoid carcinoma of the
    eyelid (PHCE) 192, *193*
progressive staining 78
proliferations of the mantle area *103*
prospect theory 11
punch biopsy 36

R
reconstruction, in MMS 22
regressive staining 78
risk stratification
  of BCC 95–102
  of cSCC 114–119
  depth of invasion 100
  histopathology 95–102
  patient factors 102
  perineural invasion 100, *101,* 119, *120, 122*
  primary versus recurrence 102
  site 100

S
safety margins 50, *50,* 124, *126,* 176, *226*
sarcomatoid BCC *99*
sarcomatoid differentiation *116*
sebaceous apparatus *103*
sebaceous carcinoma 184–187, *186–187*
serial transverse vertical cross-sections 54–59
sfumato technique 148
shave biopsy 36, *37, 38,* 129
sialometaplasia 124
slide preparation 77–78, **79**
slow Mohs 6, 15, **16**
smartphone WSI *14*
Sox-10 85, 142, **144**
spaghetti technique 132, 196, *196*
specimen preparation
  bread loaf technique 54–59, *55–57, 58,* **59**
  debulk considerations 70
  en face 3D technique 66–69, *67, 68,* **69,** *69*

hybrid technique 132, *133*
inking 53–54, *54*
in MMS 22, *23, 24*
Mohs technique 59–66, *59–65,* **66,** *66*
Munich technique 69, *69,* **70**
orientation 53, *207*
perimeter techique **70**
perimeter technique 70
peripheral sectioning of wedge excisions 70, **71,** *71*
processing issues 71–75, *74*
safety margins 71, *72–73*
serial transverse vertical cross-sections 54–59
spaghetti technique 132, 196, *196*
square technique 132, *133*
techniques 54–70, 132
spindle cell tumor 153, *154–155,* 224
squamous cell carcinoma (SCC) 18
  high-risk features **31**
  immunohistochemistry 86
  indication guidelines for MCS 31
  and MCC *170*
  very high-risk features **32**
square technique 132, *133*
staining
  AE1/AE3 86
  CK5/6 86
  common problems with rapid HE **79,** *79–83*
  fixation 78
  hemotoxylin and eosin 77–78, **78**
  p63/p40 86, *87*
  practical tips **79**
  toluidine blue stain 77
standard ring first level 42, *42*
starburst giant cells **140**
superficial BCC 92, *93*
surgical margin
  assessment xix
  definition xvii
surgical procedure 21–22
surgical techniques
  biopsy 36–38
  clinical marking 38–39, *39*
  debulk 38
  depth of excision 42, *43*
  levels 39, 40–41, *40*
  mapping 39–40, *40*
  nontargeted resections 45, *46*
  targeted resections 45, 46, *46*
sutures 55
syringoma 180, *181*
syringometaplasia 124, *125*

T

targeted resections 45, 46, *46*
telepathology 6, 13–14, *15*, 144
Thinking, Fast and Slow (Kahneman) 29
tissue preservation 21
tissue sparing 41, 51, *51*
toluidine blue stain 77
training, for MMS 22–24
trichilemmoma *106*
trichoblastoma *105*
trichoepithelioma *105*
trichofolliculoma *104*
Tübinger Muffin technique 67, *68*
Tübinger Torte technique 67, *68*
tumor size 47, *48*

U

UICC. *See* Union for International Cancer Control
    (UICC)
undifferentiated Sarcoma 231
Union for International Cancer Control (UICC) 33

V

vascular invasion *119*
volcanoes xvii–xix, *xviii–xix*

W

wedge excisions 70, **71**, *71*
whole slide imaging (WSI) 13, *13*, *14*
wide local excision (WLE)
    compared with MCS 92
    compared with MMS 19, 20–21
WSI. *See* whole slide imaging (WSI)

Z

ZnCL2 5